MARIA OAK R.G.N. SAVE THE CHILDREN.

THE smallest ENEMY

THE smallest ENEMY

understanding and avoiding infection

Dr Roy Pilsworth

Grey Seal London

First published 1990 by *Grey Seal Books*
28 Burgoyne Road, London N4 1AD, England

British Library Cataloguing in Publication
Pilsworth, Roy
The smallest enemy.
1. Man. Communicable diseases
I. Title
616.9
ISBN 1-85640-008-5

Dedicated to the memory of
Sir Graham Selby Wilson ('G.S.')
The Last Bacteriologist

The smallest enemies of mankind are the tiny living creatures that invade his body and cause him distress.

If kept at arm's length many of them are amusing fellows but without an atom of virtue; perhaps therein lies their fascination for me.

Dr Roy Pilsworth continued his education during World War II, leaving St Mary's Hospital Medical School, London, in 1942 as a Member of the Royal College of Surgeons and a Licentiate of the Royal College of Physicians, and in 1943 as a Bachelor of Surgery and a *Medicine Baccalaureus*. He joined the Public Health Laboratory Service in 1945, obtained the Diploma in Bacteriology from London University (with distinction) in 1947, and fulfilled his national service requirements in the U.K., Egypt and East Africa in 1948–50. He returned to the Public Health Laboratory Service in 1950 as Director of the Southend Laboratory, then moved to a newly built laboratory in Chelmsford in 1956, where he worked until retirement in 1983. During the last ten years at Chelmsford, he ran, with the able assistance of Mrs Pilsworth, a regional virus laboratory involved mainly in trying to prevent congenital handicaps in children born to mothers who had been infected during pregnancy.

Dr and Mrs Pilsworth have one daughter who is married to an MP and two grandchildren. While happily retired to South Benfleet, Essex, Dr Pilsworth continues his interest in writing, travelling, painting, photography, and watching rugby football and opera films.

Contents

Introduction

Books are strange animals; they undergo a process of evolution even during their period of gestation. This book was originally designed as a sort of catharsis. A method of getting out of my system the accumulated (and often disjointed) recollections of a lifetime spent in the field of microbiology. Perhaps I hoped to 'spring clean' my mind in order to adopt another, nearly as interesting, subject for the remainder of my life.

At this time I had already decided on its approximate structure and this was one that would serve as an introduction to the subject of infection for those readers without a medical or scientific background. I would not wish to appear patronizing in this endeavour—indeed, as a medical student I usually found it profitable to read nonscientific but readable accounts of a given subject before proceeding to the orthodox textbook; many of the works of René Dubos I found excellent stepping stones to help me to more structured works of science and it was a popular book *Bacteriology*, published in the Home University Library series and written by Professor Carl Browning of the University of Glasgow, that first aroused my interest in the subject at the age of fifteen.

Thus the book was already wearing two hats, but it seemed too good not to miss the opportunity of trying to include a few basic rules for the avoidance of the various infections. I hope this will not suggest that this is a 'do-it-yourself-and-call-in-the-doctor-when-moribund' type of book. When infection seems likely medical advice should always be sought, but it is far more important to avoid an infection than to cure one, so that a little common-sense advice has been included in most chapters.

As if this were not enough, what struck me while getting together the notes for this book was the vast difference between infection in the West and that in poorer countries, euphemistically described as the Third World, developing countries and so on. This difference seemed to me one based on money and organization. The Industrial Revolution had been a Western phenomenon and, in the days of imperialism, it had been in the interests of the West to prevent it from occurring in the poorer countries in order to maintain adequate markets for Western goods. However, not only money seemed to be concerned, although this was the most important matter, but also organization, wars, graft, nepotism and racism (and we have to remember that there is a considerable amount of racism outside South Africa, usually described as tribalism), all highly efficient methods of squandering money, food, services and lives. Thus the impact of infection in the Third World is incompletely understood by many workers in Western countries and the burden of it in the West is so comparatively light that we ought to try to remove the beam in our brother's eye before we bother with the mote in our own.

Finally, having found a publisher brave enough to consider publishing the book, I was persuaded to attempt to project my feelings and experiences in the matter of infection into the future as far as I could. It is well known that the only really safe prediction that one can make is that life is unpredictable, so that this section of the book is likely to be quite unreliable as an accurate guide to the future. However, if it stimulates or enrages others so much that they form their own views on the matter, it will have served its purpose.

This should be a good season for writing books about infection because, in the West, there has never been so much public interest in it since the days of the Black Death. This is not because of any real increase in the importance on the whole of infection but, I believe, because of the affluent circumstances in which we live there is greater leisure for thinking about the matter, the minds of most people not being preoccupied by thoughts of penury or war. An added reason is the efficiency of the media in reporting (and usually over-emphasizing the importance) of illness and handicap of all kinds. Because, unlike trauma or cancer, infectious processes are self-perpetuating, they give reporters a longer run for their money.

It might be thought worthwhile to consider a few of the infectious diseases that have brought headaches to politicians and a living to medical journalists over the last year or so.

Aids. Perhaps the most frightening epidemic to appear since the introduction of syphilis in the fifteenth century is the Acquired Immune Deficiency Syndrome (AIDS). One of its greatest powers for causing alarm is our ignorance of how it will progress and, in spite of modern scientific methods, we are very much in the situation of a population exposed to plague during the Middle Ages. We have not, so far, burned any Jews over the matter, as was then done, but an unusual strength of prejudice has been directed against sufferers from the disease and also serious suggestions made that the virus was synthesized in the Soviet Union and released in the Western countries!

Rumours and rumours of rumours have flitted across the pages and screens, discussed at high levels by scientific and medical bodies, their deliberations translated into the language of the gutter in order that those at greatest risk may understand a situation not completely comprehended by their more intelligent peers; this has resulted in a state of chaos, with those hardly at risk in a state of panic and those most at risk confidently unaware of the fact. However, recent reports suggest that the correct counsels are being heeded, limited though their value may be. Some of the political infighting over the detection of the AIDS virus is described in the text.

Cryptosporidiosis. This condition has not often made the headlines because it is a long word and difficult to spell. It is a newly described disease in humans but has already had a few moments of glory; it is caused by a small parasite which gives rise to diarrhoea, mainly in infants, and usually of a mild variety. It has been found in drinking water supplies (once in company with another parasite, *Giardia lamblia*) and its name would seem more fearsome than its effects although its elimination is certainly desirable.

Hepatitis B. It was shown in 1965 that there were at least two distinct forms of virus commonly causing liver infection, a fact that had been suspected since the 1930s. This explained why people receiving blood transfusions occasionally developed jaundice afterwards and also supplied a means of eliminating batches of blood containing the virus. As a result (and to avoid litigation) the Government immediately spent vast sums of money equipping blood transfusion centres in Britain with fully equipped and staffed virus laboratories. The experience gained has turned out to be useful in eliminating the AIDS virus from blood also.

Influenza. This infection has not received much publicity recently, but I feel sure it will do so again, in due time. However, it is to be hoped that vaccination will successfully repel infection by any of the present strains and that a new vaccine will rapidly be made if a new strain of the virus emerges.

Legionnaire's disease. This infection, named from the 1976 outbreak in Philadelphia, continues to plague hospitals and cities, causing quite large outbreaks and quite a few deaths. It would seem that the use of wet cooling towers and certain forms of air conditioning should either be regularly monitored or banned completely.

Listeria infection. A rare infection that causes very few deaths, listeria does, however, cause *some* deaths and should be eliminated if possible. This sort of condition raises the question of priorities, always present in medicine; should one carry out one heart replacement or repair large numbers of hernias for the same price? Deaths from listeria infection most frequently occur in patients suffering from other medical conditions as well. As salmonella infections (see below) cause more deaths, mainly in the otherwise ill and old, should we address ourselves to the more important salmonella question before getting too excited about listeria?

Rubella. The risk of a child being born with congenital disabilities because its mother contracted rubella during pregnancy has hardly altered since the condition was recognized some forty years ago. From time to time the Department of Health has organized campaigns intended to bring forward women susceptible to infection so that they can be vaccinated. The force of most such campaigns appeared to be completely dissipated by the time they had reached the consumer; following the announcement of one such campaign, our laboratories were given extra money to fund the extra work expected; in reality we had slightly fewer tests to carry out during the following year. The new practice of giving a combined measles - mumps - rubella vaccine during the early years of life should improve the future situation considerably.

Salmonella infections. Salmonella infections have been with us for a long time. The greatest risks are from raw meat, poultry and made-up food not intended to be further cooked. For years the danger of duck eggs causing salmonella infection has been recognized; their danger arises from the duck's ovaries being infected so that the egg is infected within the shell. Now the same thing appears to be happening to eggs from chickens. Only a minute proportion of eggs on the market are infected in this way; nevertheless, to avoid the small risk of infection it is important that all eggs should be well cooked before consumption. This is unfortunate for those who like their bread-and-butter 'soldiers'!

I should add yet another reason for writing this book, perhaps the most important. Stories about outbreaks of infection, about the devious paths that infecting organisms take in order to multiply their kind, about the heroic deaths suffered by some seekers after the truth in these matters, how some people have profited by the pestilences of others—all these make a very good read. Infection involves both the greatness and littleness of mankind and the gentleness and simplicity that are perhaps best exemplified in the case of the man who developed psittacosis because he gave his ailing budgerigar the kiss of life!

ONE

A Definition of Infection

One of the minor atrocities committed during the Second World War was the invention of the Brains Trust. This consisted of a handful of knowledgeable (or eminent) men (mainly) who tried to enlighten or amuse their audiences by attempting to answer questions on any subject, whether or not it was within their spheres of knowledge. One of the most successful stars of this programme was Professor C.E.M. Joad, a philosopher and psychologist. It was his habit, before attempting to answer a question, to make sure that both he and his audience invested with the same meaning the words and phrases used in the question. His opening remark was usually 'It depends what you mean by . . .'. He had realized that, once the terms used had been strictly defined, a great amount of confusion could be avoided. A definition of terms at the outset has spoiled many good rows in politics, science and religion. We have to imitate Professor Joad and define exactly what we mean by the word 'infection'.

Definition of infection

A good definition seems to be 'The invasion of the body by other living creatures that are capable of causing illness as a result'. However, there are two small inconsistencies to note in this definition. The body normally contains many living organisms that are not capable of causing illness (as long as they remain in the part of the body where they normally live), and many organisms that *are* capable of causing illness do *not* do so for various reasons.

Organisms normally present in the human body

The normal body contains a large variety of harmless organisms and although these are mainly very small in size, there are at least two varieties of larger organisms – mites – found in it. One variety lives in the eyelashes and, although it looks ferocious under the microscope, it is quite harmless. It does not seem to have any purpose in life, but a colleague of mine insists that it is present to curb inordinate pride. 'Next time,' he says, 'you are harangued from the television screen by a self-appointed guardian of public morals, look her straight in the eyelashes and remember that, even as she is speaking, there are mites in them actively copulating!'

However, it is in the digestive tract that most organisms are to be found. (See Figure 1.1.) The mouth, for instance, contains many harmless organisms, which together with organisms present in food are constantly being swallowed. But the stomach, because it produces strong hydrochloric acid which is lethal to most organisms, remains practically sterile (this is a powerful defence against food-borne infection). As we pass down the alimentary canal, organisms occur in greater and greater numbers so that in the stools, the solid waste passed each day (by the regular person), there may be as many as 10,000,000,000 organisms in each gram of solid waste.

Figure 1.1 Numbers of bacteria in the alimentary tract

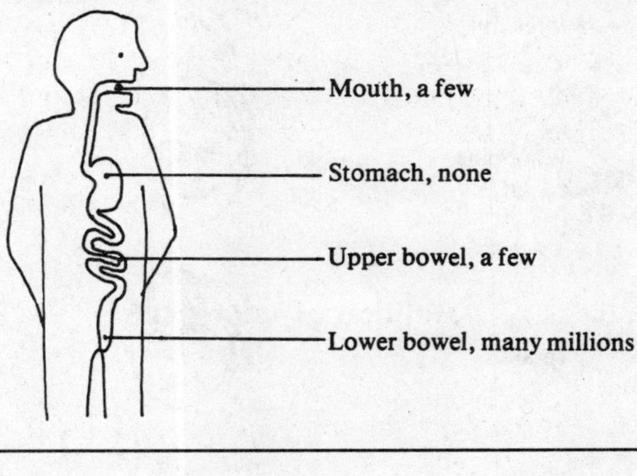

Ruminant animals, such as cattle and horses, carry even greater numbers of organisms in the intestinal tract; these animals live almost entirely on grass which, when intact, is not a very promising source of energy. However, the organisms within the ruminant are able to break down the cellulose that it contains into sugars. The stomach of the horse is one vast fermenting vat where this occurs and the animal uses the sugars produced directly for energy production. The situation is very like the changing of sugar into alcohol by yeast in the production of beer, except that, in the case of the horse, the process goes on inside the consumer, while, so far, no one has yet devised a system of internal brewing for man!

Organisms that can cause illness do not always do so

When a person develops an infection such as rubella, or is vaccinated against such an infection, antibodies are formed. These are proteins of a special sort that appear in the blood and whose job it is to prevent further infections by *that organism* should it appear again. These substances are specific; that is, vaccination against whooping cough will protect against whooping cough only and vaccination against tetanus against tetanus only. (See Figure 1.2.) Antibodies can be detected in the blood of patients and their presence indicates that the person has either suffered from the disease in the past or has been vaccinated against it. The detection of such antibodies is a useful way of determining how common a certain infectious disease is in a community. Below is an

Figure 1.2 Vaccination is specific

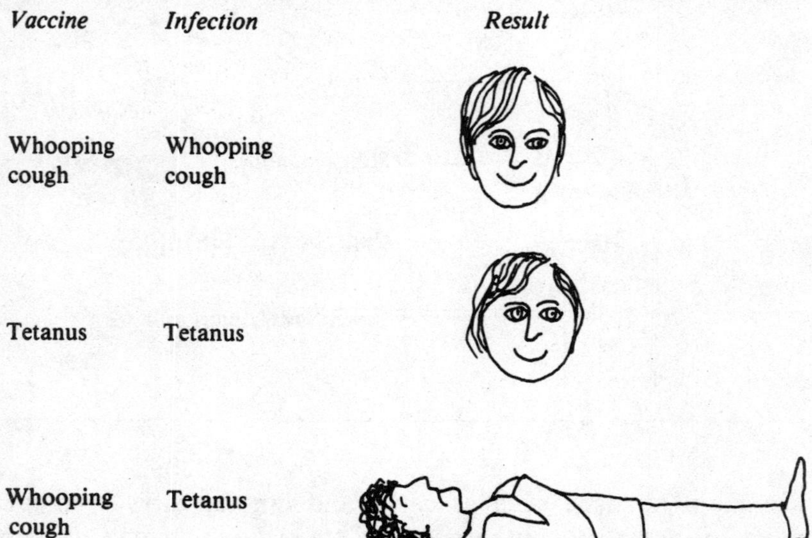

example which also includes indications that patients are sometimes not reliable witnesses.

German measles in boys

Suppose we are interested in the importance of German measles (rubella) in the community; if we take blood from 100 boys when they leave school and look for antibodies to rubella, we may find that fifty of the boys have such antibodies, showing that these fifty have had the disease at some time or other (boys are not vaccinated against rubella so that the antibodies will not have appeared as a result of vaccination). If, before the blood was taken, each boy was given a form to indicate what illness he had suffered from, we should probably discover that, of the fifty boys with antibody, only about twenty-five remembered having had German measles. Thus twenty-five had the disease without knowing about it—that is, subclinically.

Of the boys without antibody, four or five may remember having had rubella—as they have no antibody they cannot have had the infection! This shows how unreliable is the diagnosis of rubella in the absence of blood tests (quite often a mother will object to her daughter being vaccinated against rubella on the grounds that she has already had the disease. In about 25 per cent of these cases the diagnosis will have been incorrect and the girl is still likely to contract the disease if not vaccinated).

Thus infection can occur without causing illness and, when pregnant women develop rubella infections that harm their babies, in 50 per cent of cases the infection will have occurred without their knowledge. Even fewer cases of actual illness follow infection by the poliomyelitis virus and many other infective agents. (See Figure 1.3.)

Figure 1.3 Infection does not always produce illness—in poliomyelitis, for instance, when one hundred are infected

So we have to define infection as an invasion of the body by organisms *capable* of causing illness but which do not *always* do so.

Infection and inflammation

These two conditions are sometimes confused. Inflammation is one of the body's reactions to damage of any kind and it may be caused by infection or by burns, cuts and scratches, blows, sensitivity reactions and many other sorts of injury. Although most people can usually recognize inflammation fairly easily, earlier physicians described the five cardinal signs of it to help the less perceptive:

Tumor – swelling
Calor – affected part feels warm
Dolor – pain
Rubor – redness over the affected region
Loss of use – if a limb is affected it becomes difficult to use

The basic change in the tissues that occurs in inflammation is a widening of the blood vessels in the affected area. This allows more blood to reach the inflamed part and, because the walls of the blood vessels are stretched, they become thin and allow fluid and cells to leak through.

This increase of fluid – which causes the pain and swelling – has the effect of diluting any poison that might have been produced locally (either from bacteria or some of the body's own damaged cells) and washes away the damaged cells and their products. At the same time there is an increase in the number of white cells arriving at the site; these kill and devour any bacteria present and also carry away debris (when these white cells accumulate in large numbers they form pus; see chapter three). Thus the effects of inflammation resemble the management of an accident on a motorway: first the area is hosed to remove toxic substances and then lorries arrive to take away the debris. In both cases – much later on – repairs to the fabric are carried out. (See Figure 1.4.)

Organisms that cause infection

A start in life

Scientists are understandably reticent about speculating upon the origin of life on Earth, but, if pressed, they will proceed somewhat as follows.

Millions of years ago the seas were still warm and contained high concentrations of ammonia, methane and carbon dioxide. They were also subject to constant bombardment by electrical storms. As a result a variety of molecules were formed of varying degrees of complexity. Laboratory experiments, using a few litres of water containing what was believed to be present in the primeval ocean and then bombarded with electrical discharges, have produced, after a short period of treatment, quite complicated molecules of the sort that go to making living things. (See Figure 1.5a.)

Figure 1.4 Changes during inflammation

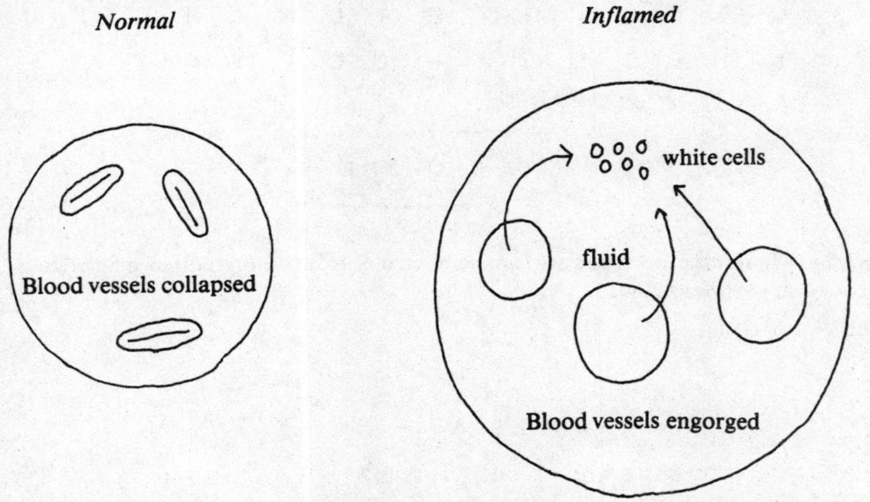

Thus the best theory, but still an odds against one, is that, in the enormous time and volume of water involved, there appeared a complicated molecule capable of reproducing itself.

A lot of philosophical nonsense has been written about Life as if it were a concept that the average person could not grasp. There is no difficulty; deciding where life starts is simply a question of defining what, to a practical mind, life consists of. I would suggest that, at its simplest, life consists of the ability of a fairly complicated molecule to abstract substances from its environment and thus grow and finally to give rise to further molecules closely resembling itself.

Accepting this definition, the first life to emerge was in the form of a long molecule which was able to increase its size by removing substances from the 'primeval soup' in the oceans of that time. (See

Figure 1.5 The origin of life

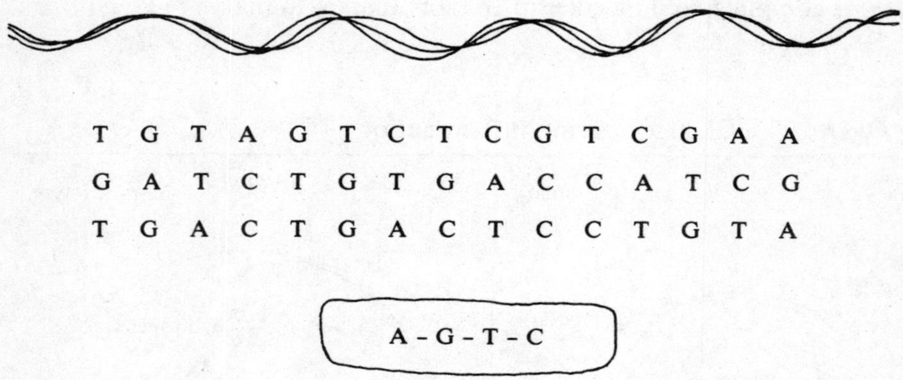

1.5a Many large molecules are formed by chance from the myriads of smaller ones in the primeval sea.

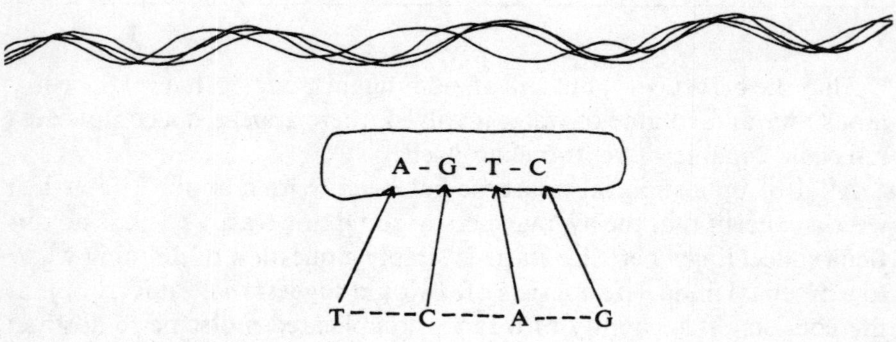

1.5b Other small molecules from the environment become attached to their opposite numbers on the large molecule so that a large double molecule is formed. Ts and As join together, as do Cs and Gs.

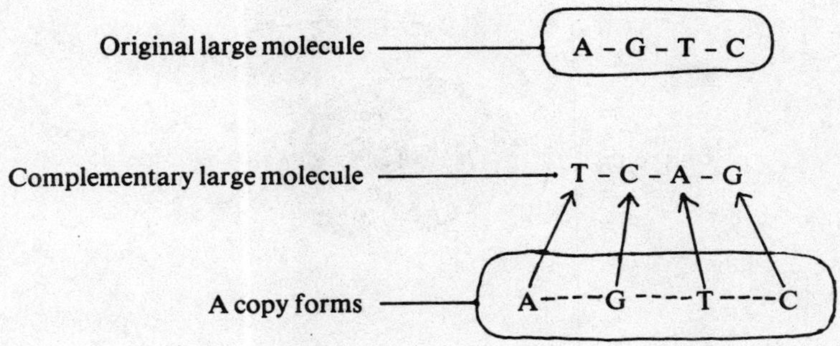

1.5c The process is repeated and small molecules become attached to the complementary large molecule, providing an exact copy of the original large molecule.

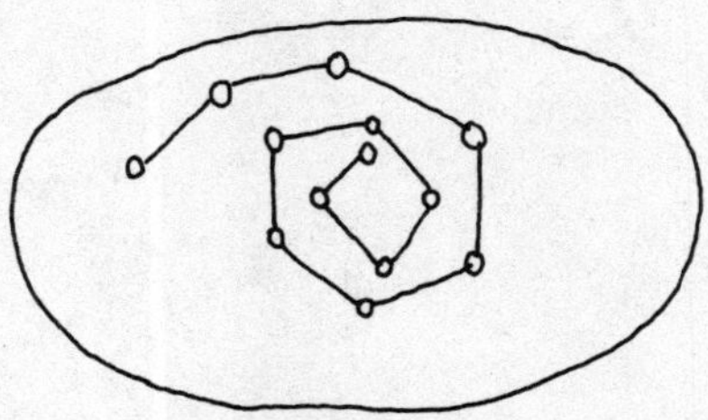

1.5d The large molecule becomes longer and more complex and develops a membrane to provide it with its own environment and to protect it.

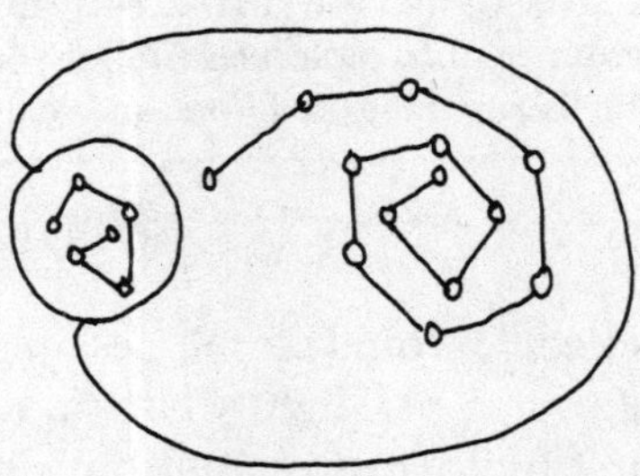

1.5e *Predators have arrived*. There is now a large variety of large molecules and some have learned how to save time and energy by destroying their fellows and using the latter's small molecules to build their own cells.

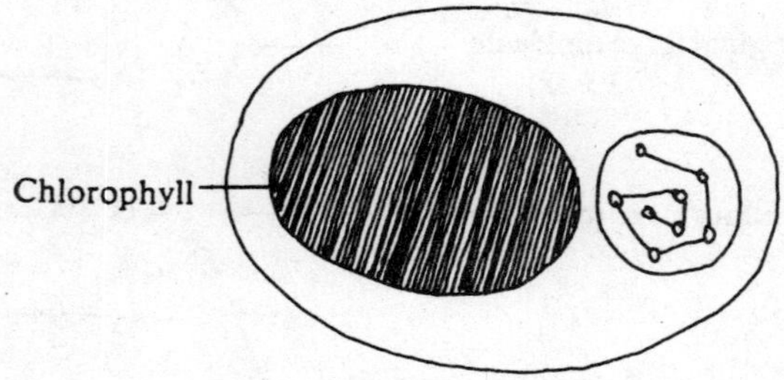

1.5f *Life now really takes off*. Chlorophyll appears and green plants can now use the sun's energy to make the small molecules formerly obtained from the environment by sheer luck.

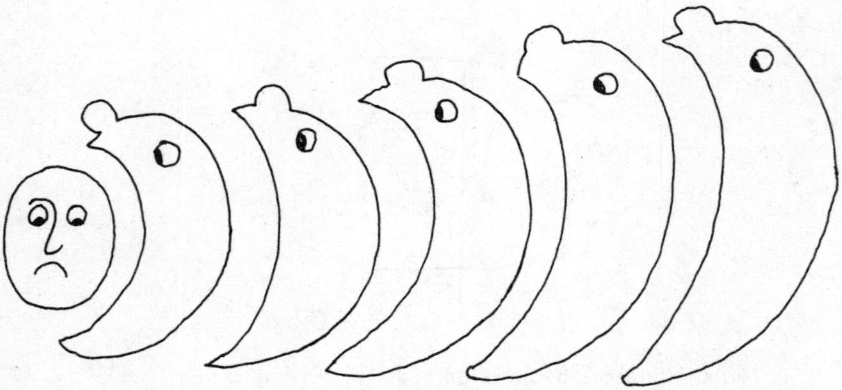

1.5g Predators now develop on a grand scale to harvest plant life and thus bypass the need to scrounge small molecules from the environment. Further predators develop that live on these predators, and so on *ad infinitum*.

Figure 1.5 b&c.) This molecule would closely resemble the chromosomes of the living creatures of today, or, slightly later in its development, *simple viruses*. Thus the first biological revolution was the appearance of something we can call life.

It is unlikely that our molecule was the first to approach the ability to reproduce; it is probable that millions of similar molecules fell at the last ditch. However, it is probable that *only one such molecule gave rise to living things*. This statement is based on the fact that all living things possess, along their chromosomes, only four substances used for containing information (with occasional slight variation). This strongly suggests that our molecule possessed these same four substances—guanine, thymine, adenine and cytosine (G, T, A and C).

The next stage of evolution was the emergence of the cell. Our primeval molecule was at the mercy of changes in the temperature and the acidity or alkalinity of its environment. At some stage in its history, this primeval molecule succeeded in putting a wall around itself to protect it from a hostile environment and to preserve for it continually the environment that it thrived in best. (See Figure 1.5d.) At this stage the molecule grew more complex and became coiled up in the centre of its 'mini-environment', thus becoming what we call a nucleus.

Our molecule had now become a quite complex affair, *resembling a bacterium by today's classification*. Its cell also gave it a new-found freedom and this led to the second biological revolution. Certain strains of our molecule (now our cell) found that there were more efficient ways of surviving than depending upon the fortuitous presence of suitable growth molecules in their environment; they found it quicker and more efficient to use ready-made compounds that had been produced by other organisms from simple substances; thus the new cells started with quite complicated molecules and were able to produce their own substances much more rapidly. (See Figure 1.5e.) Hence the first predators appeared and initiated a practice that has been copied by all the higher organisms, especially Man.

While life depended upon the fortuitous presence of useful molecules in the environment, its pace of development was very slow, but a remarkable degree of acceleration of this pace followed the emergence of the green pigment, chlorophyll, which enabled the cell to trap some of the enormous output of energy of the sun. Thus there emerged a group of cells that did not need to use either their immediate environment or their neighbours to produce energy and to build further cell material. In this way the plant world emerged and from that point life really took off. (See Figure 1.5f.) Not only were green cells able to multiply at an enormous rate compared with the previous almost stationary condition, but soon the other cells found that they could use the material of the green cells for their own growth—these were the first animals. In addition, further groups of 'animals' fed off the animals that ate the 'plants'; then other groups fed on these further groups and so on *ad infinitum* so that soon complex food chains evolved like those that exist in nature today. (See Figure 1.5g.)

In a manner something like this, those organisms that cause infections to larger creatures evolved. The types of organisms that cause infection are:

Organisms	*Examples of infection*
Viruses	Rubella
Bacteria	Scarlet fever
Fungi	Ringworm
Single celled parasites	Malaria
Worms	Threadworm
Arthropods (creatures like insects)	Scabies

The sizes of organisms

Before talking about the sizes of organisms we have to decide on the units we are going to use – because of the small size of our organisms we have to use very small units. (See Figure 1.6.) In the big world the metre is the commonest unit of length – about 39 inches. To give us a more suitable unit we divide this by 1,000,000 to give what is called a micrometre (μm) – about 1/25,000 of an inch.

Most bacteria are about 1 μm thick and either spherical or 4–5 μm long.

For viruses we need an even smaller unit so we divide a micrometre by 1000 and call it a nanometre (nm). This is about 1/25,000,000 in and small viruses may be as small as 20 nm (about a millionth of an inch) in diameter while large ones will be about 500 nm in diameter.

Figure 1.6 Sizes of organisms

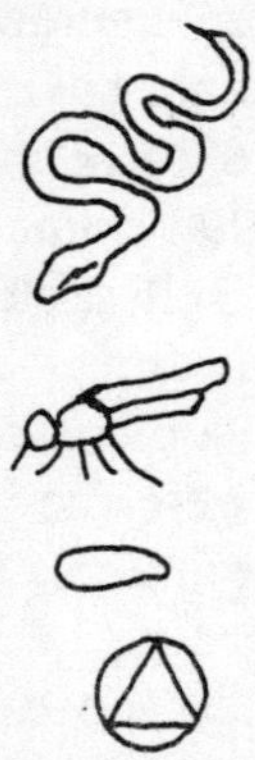

Snake is 1 m

Insect is 10 mm

Bacterium is 1 μm × 4–5 μm

Virus is 20–500 nm

1 metre (m)
1,000 millimetres (mm)
1,000,000 micrometres (μm)
1,000,000,000 nanometres (nm)

Viruses

We shall talk about the structure of viruses when talking about genetics and infection. Viruses are common causes of infection and, because of their behaviour, they can be said to be totally harmful as a group; their only possible use to man is in the control of pests and even in these situations they are not always successful. The main properties of viruses are:

1. They are so small in size that they cannot be seen with a conventional microscope and are able to pass through filters which will hold back bacteria. (See Figure 1.7.)

Figure 1.7 Viruses can pass through filters that hold back bacteria

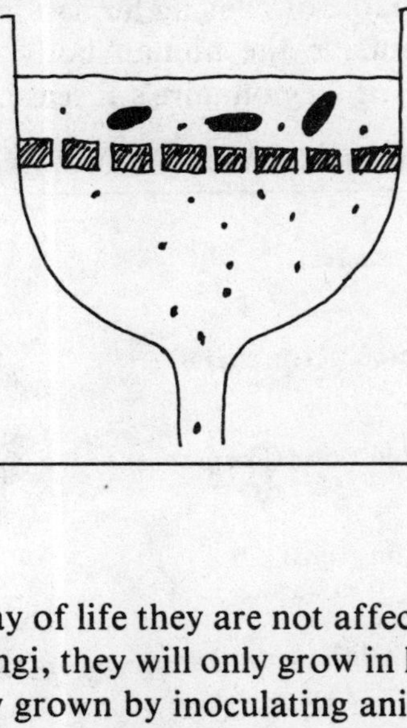

2. Because of their way of life they are not affected by antibiotics and, unlike bacteria and fungi, they will only grow in living cells. In the early days they were usually grown by inoculating animals but this was both expensive and unreliable—although chimps developed poliomyelitis, many human viruses infect humans only and cannot infect animals.
3. In 1946 it was found that viruses would grow in tissue culture—that is, human or monkey cells grown on the walls of test tubes. This is not an easy method but has been developed over the last forty years and is today the main method of growing and identifying viruses.

Many human diseases are caused by viruses and no doubt more will be discovered in the future. Some of the better known are:

AIDS
Chickenpox
Cytomegalovirus
Glandular fever
Hepatitis A and B
Herpes
Lassa fever
Measles
Mumps
Pneumonia
Poliomyelitis
Psittacosis
Rabies
Rubella
Shingles
Smallpox

Bacteria

These are usually thought of as being minute plants. However they do not possess the green pigment chlorophyll so that they cannot obtain their energy from sunlight and have to rely on food already made by other organisms. Many live on dead animal and vegetable matter and others live on the scraps they can pick up in some of the body orifices of animals but without causing illness. Of the thousands of different sorts of bacteria only a hundred or so cause harm to man and most of these flourish mainly in the human body, being passed from patient to patient either directly or through food etc. or via a carrier. Only a few common organisms capable of causing human infection can thrive and multiply indefinitely outside the human body and these include the bacterium responsible for Legionnaire's disease.

Figure 1.8 Shapes and arrangements of some bacteria

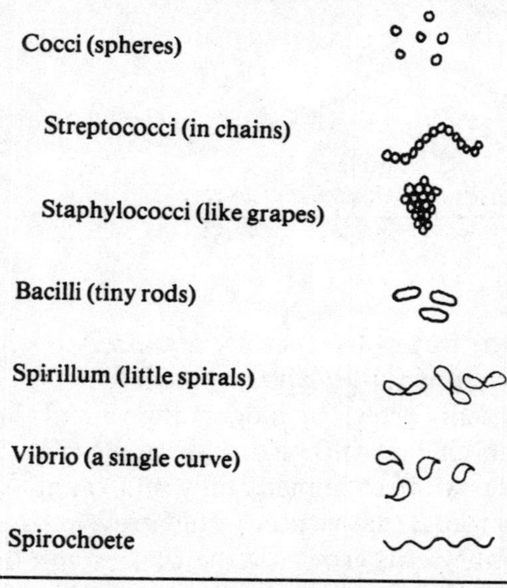

Bacteria are larger than viruses and can be seen with an ordinary (light) microscope. They are usually either spherical or sausage shaped. (See Figure 1.8.) The spheres are usually about 1 μm in diameter and the rods may range from 2 or 3 μm to long threads many microns in length. Some are actively motile which may help their spread in the body, although this is not essential because the various body fluids in which bacteria multiply when they cause infection are constantly on the move and any organisms present are spread rapidly throughout the tissues.

An important characteristic of bacteria from the laboratory point of view is that they can be grown on simple substances – known as media; thus, when a mould grows on the surface of jam, the jam is the medium used by the mould to support growth. If bacteria are grown in liquid media, such as broth, they grow throughout the liquid, making it cloudy if sufficient organisms develop.

If the medium is made solid, using gelatin or (better still) agar, then the bacteria cannot move about and they grow in little heaps that get bigger as the organisms multiply. These heaps are called colonies and they are important because the main way that bacteria are first identified is by the appearance of the colony.

Although bacteria can only be seen individually by using a microscope and laboratories are usually associated in the lay mind with microscopes, the latter are relatively rarely used when dealing with bacteria. The appearance of the colony and the determination of which substances (usually sugars) that the organism can break down are usually sufficient to identify it.

Diseases caused by bacteria include:

Anthrax	Impetigo
Boils and abscesses	Legionnaire's disease
Botulism	Meningitis
Brucellosis	Plague
Diarrhoea	Pneumonia
Diphtheria	Scarlet fever
Dysentery	Tetanus
Food poisoning	Typhoid fever
Hospital infections	Whooping cough

Fungi

When compared with viruses and bacteria, the fungi and other causes of infection are not very important in the West. Fungi are closely related to the bacteria and also to those fungi we meet in nature – mushrooms, toadstools, etc. These are the big fungi but infection is caused by the microscopic ones. We all harbour a variety of fungi on our skin and, given the correct conditions such as the presence of soggy, unwashed feet, the fungi can penetrate the skin and cause infection. In nature, fungi perform many useful scavenging functions, one of which is to deal with desquamated skin cells shed from the human body and it has been said that, in the absence of such organisms, we might be walking ankle deep in shed human skin cells! Like bacteria fungi can be easily grown in the laboratory. They grow slowly and their colonial appearance is used for identification.

The commonest fungus infections in Britain are:

Athlete's foot
Thrush of the mouth or vagina
Ringworm
Meningitis (rarely)

Single celled parasites

These, which I will call just 'parasites' most of the time, have been thought of as being single celled animals. There are not many types of importance in this country but in the Third World they are a very important cause of illness. These organisms can usually be recognized under a microscope because their appearances are often characteristic. (See Figure 1.9.) Many can be grown in the laboratory, but usually for

Figure 1.9 Some single celled parasites

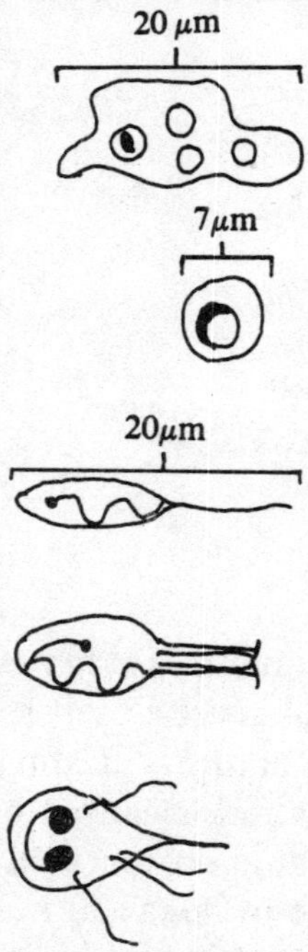

Entamoeba histolytica	Dysentery
Malarial parasite within red cell	Malaria
Trypanosome	Sleeping sickness
Trichomonas	Vaginal discharge
Giardia lamblia	Diarrhoea

research purposes rather than diagnosis. The commonest protozoal infections in Britain are:

Cryptosporidium (diarrhoea)
Trichomonas vaginalis (vaginitis)
Giardia lamblia (diarrhoea)

Giardia lamblia also affects travellers returning from Leningrad, Egypt and certain other places overseas. Other common overseas infections caused by parasites are:

Malaria
Sleeping sickness
Tropical ulcers
Amoebic dysentery

These diseases are occasionally introduced into Britain.

Worms

This group of organisms includes some of the largest parasites known. The human tapeworm, for instance, may measure up to 10 metres in length. At the other end of the scale are the minute microfilaria which can be seen only under the microscope and which can be easily transmitted by mosquitoes.

Worms tend to occur most commonly in the Third World and especially in the tropics, where they are responsible for much chronic ill health. The only common worm in the West is the pinworm or threadworm; even tapeworms are rare today. Elsewhere the following worms among others occur:

Tapeworms and Hydatid cysts
Liver flukes
Bilharzia (Schistosomiasis)
Hookworm
Onchocerciasis (River blindness)
Ascaris lumbricoides
Filarial worms (Elephantiasis)

Arthropods

These are literally 'the animals with jointed legs'—that is, the insects, spiders, mites, etc. Their main importance is in the spread of other infective diseases such as malaria, yellow fever, filarial worms, etc. However, some arthropods are offensive to man in their own right:

Scabies mite
Fleas
Head and body lice
Bedbugs
Scorpions
Spiders

Genetics and infection

Genetics is the study of the way in which characters are inherited and the shortest lesson in genetics is: 'Mary had a little lamb—the doctor *was* surprised!' We take it for granted that like gives rise to like—we have children resembling humans, cats have kittens and dogs have puppies. There are accounts of women giving birth to large numbers of chickens but these are no more believable than the suggestion made by those opposing vaccination that vaccinated women might give birth to calves!

Figure 1.10 Simple genetics

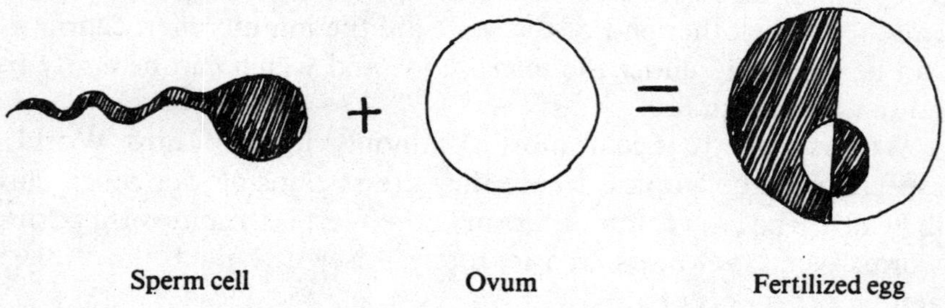

The fertilized egg contains all the information needed to build and run us all.

If we think of it, there has to be some mechanism that controls these affairs and, for instance, ensures that a child will be likely to have red hair if the mother or father has red hair also.

The whole of the body is derived ultimately from the single cell formed when the male sperm fertilizes the female egg. Thus that cell must contain all the information needed to instruct all the millions of cells of the body how to behave throughout their lifetimes and also the information that must be passed on to the next generation. (See Figure 1.10.)

Chromosomes

The information mentioned above is stored in the form of chemical substances strung along long coiled bodies known as chromosomes which reside in the nuclei of cells. (See Figure 1.11.) Those who have some knowledge of personal computers will know that information can be fed into them from ordinary audio tape cassettes in a tape player. The information is sited along the length of the chromosome just as it is along the length of a cassette tape.

Figure 1.11 The chromosome—information within the cell's nucleus

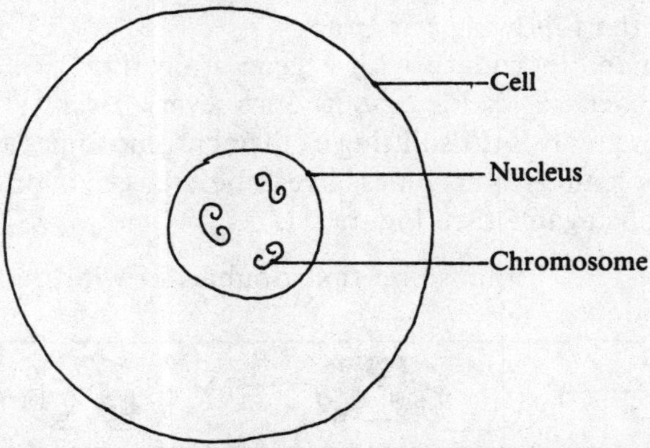

Every time a cell divides, as when the foetus grows in the womb, information is passed to both daughter cells by the chromosome splitting along its length and one half entering each of the new cells. (See Figure 1.12.) Thus, in theory, every cell of the body contains information sufficient to build and run an entire new body. This, fortunately, does not occur in humans (imagine the consequences!), but it is not

Figure 1.12 Cell, nucleus and chromosome divide together

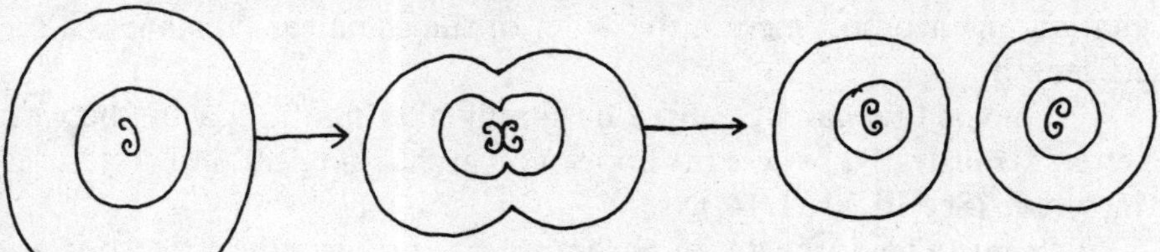

uncommon for entire new plants to develop from cuttings consisting of only a few cells.

Chromosomes and resistance to antibiotics

Chromosomes play an important part in the way that organisms are able to exploit the conditions in which they find themselves. Thirty years or so ago we believed we were entering a golden age when infection would become rare because of the newly discovered antibiotics. Disappointingly, however, many bacteria rapidly developed resistance to penicillin and other antibiotics and thus became able to grow in their presence and hence still be capable of causing infection. The way this occurs is described in the following paragraphs.

While humans reproduce with a generation time of about twenty-five years, bacteria divide about once every twenty-five minutes. Reproduction involves the splitting of their chromosomes as the bacteria divide and the split chromosomes have to be enlarged in order to be wide enough to split again. (See Figure 1.13.)

Figure 1.13 The chromosome first doubles in width and then splits down the middle

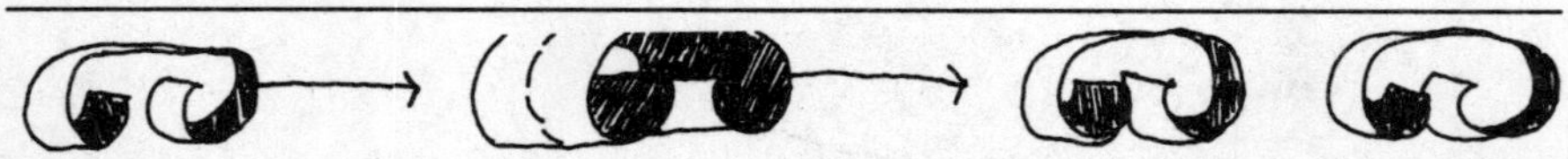

This is done by the chromosome acquiring chemical substances identical with those along its length and in exactly the same relative positions. These substances are those mentioned in the discussion on the origin of life earlier in this chapter—adenine, thymine, guanine and cytosine. These molecules, or close relatives of them, are found in the chromosomes of all living things. In most cases these substances are acquired precisely, but mistakes can happen.

If we take a simple musical tune and insert one extra note but play in the same rhythm as before we destroy the tune completely. The 'information' in the tune depends entirely on the order of notes in music, as the information in words depends on the order of letters and the information on chromosomes on the order of the chemical substances along its length.

The havoc that can be caused by simply altering the spacing between letters is illustrated, where the hope of an archaeological find was falsely inspired. (See Figure 1.14.)

Such mistakes in bacterial chromosomes are usually disastrous and the bacteria possessing them perish and are thus unable to transmit the altered chromosomes to their offspring. However, these mistakes can occasionally be of use of the organism.

To return to our writing analogy, imagine, for instance, a quite reasonable instruction on a fire extinguisher: 'To be used on fires.' This is good information in the vast majority of cases, but, if, for reasons unknown, some fire extinguishers came to be filled with petrol, the result of their use on fires would bring about disaster. Suppose again, out of many millions, one instruction was wrongly written: '*Not* to be used on fires', then the operator heeding this instruction would be preserved.

Figure 1.14 The importance of spacing

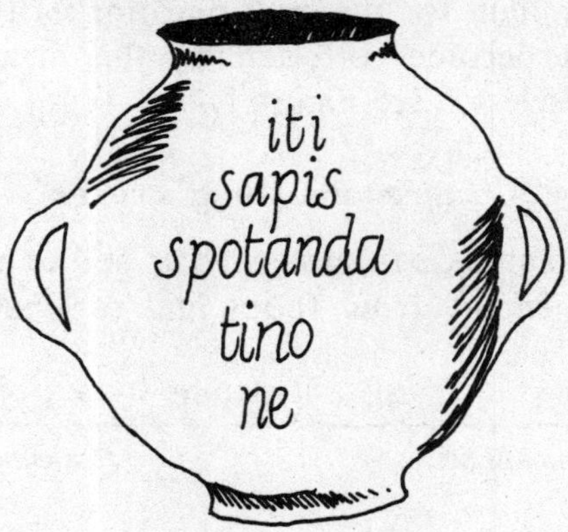

Information depends on content, order and spacing. This vessel was believed to be a valuable archaeological find until this inscription was respaced.

This kind of situation may sometimes apply to bacterial chromosomes. Suppose a strain of bacterium uses a substance A for its growth and energy mechanism. Suppose also that the effect of penicillin is to destroy substance A; when bacteria of this strain are exposed to penicillin, they will starve to death for lack of substance A. Suppose, for a third time, that, through a mistake in the chromosome development because of its acquisition of the 'wrong' chemical, one bacterium receives the altered message: 'Use substance B' then this organism will be able to multiply rapidly, partly because of the availability of substance B and partly through the lack of competition on the part of its colleagues who will have starved to death. (See Figure 1.15.)

It would seem unlikely, on the face of it, that such a helpful direction could arise by chance; however, millions and millions of cell divisions take place in a few hours in a culture of bacteria and there is scope for millions of 'mistakes' and although most of these will be lethal, the odd one that is helpful will survive because of the advantage it confers on those organisms that possess it. These bacteria will breed true giving rise to more penicillin resistant bacteria.

To give a more specific instance, a patient may be suffering from a staphylococcal infection in the form of a bone abscess. He is given penicillin which kills most of the offending bacteria but, among the huge number of cell divisions taking place, luckily for the bacterium but unluckily for the patient, there is one mutation that allows the organism to grow in the presence of penicillin. All the other bacteria present will die, leaving a clear field for the multiplication of the resistant strain. If another patient becomes infected by this strain treatment with penicillin will be useless. (See Figure 1.15.)

Chromosomes and viruses

Most animals and plants carry, within their bodies and cells, the apparatus for deriving energy from foods and for making new material

Figure 1.15 Selection of resistant strains by antibiotics

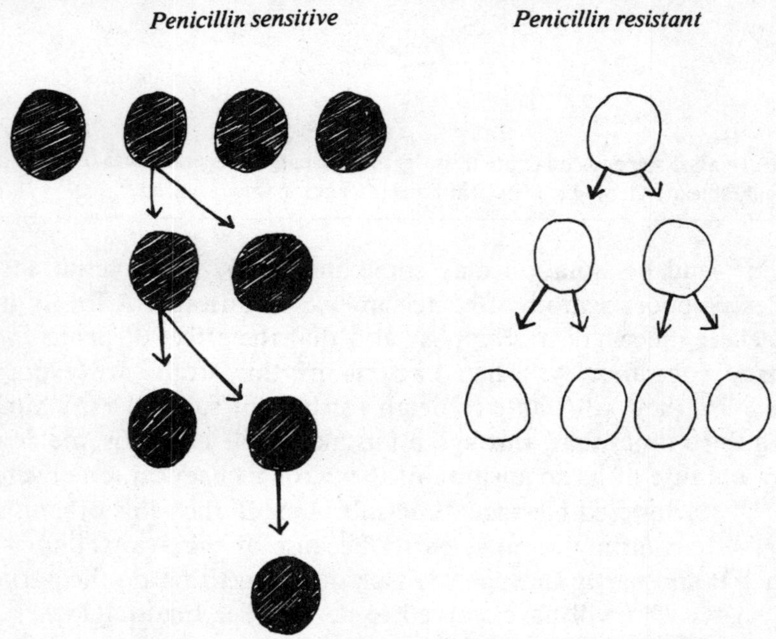

suitable for their own growth and reproduction. These mechanisms are controlled by information present in the chromosomes.

Viruses, however, have no such mechanisms; they consist almost entirely of chromosomes with usually a protein coat to protect them when they pass from cell to cell. They are so lacking in normal cell mechanisms that they depend on the cells of other organisms for their own growth and reproduction.

The substance on chromosomes that carries the information is called nucleic acid and every creature has its own peculiar make of nucleic acid (NA) as if the organism were a complicated lock and its personal NA the only key that will fit it. When a virus enters a cell (e.g. a herpes virus entering a skin cell) the NA of the virus overrides the NA in the chromosomes of the cell. This stops the cell's internal mechanism from producing 'cell material' and diverts it to producing 'virus material'. (See Figure 1.16.) In this way viruses are constructed within the cell and when

Figure 1.16 Viruses multiply only within cells

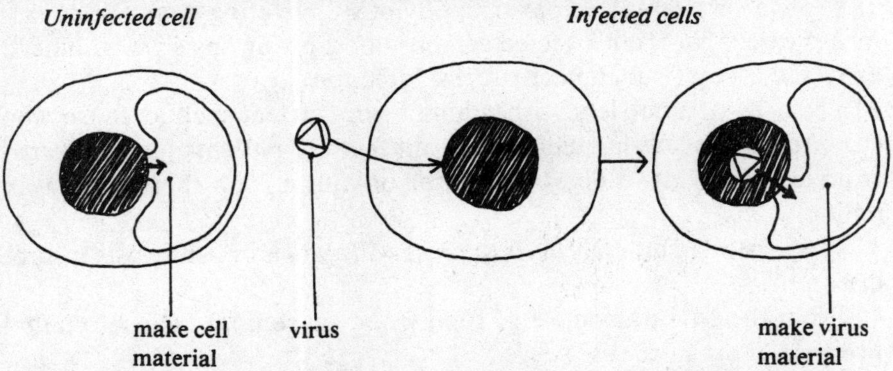

sufficient have been formed, they leave the cell to infect further cells, and like the vandals they are, cause damage as they do so. It is this damage that accounts for the symptoms of the illnesses caused by many viruses, although some well-behaved viruses can 'squat' harmlessly for years.

Most antibiotics destroy bacteria by interfering with their 'growth and reproduction' mechanisms; as viruses lack these they are unaffected by antibiotics.

TWO

How Infections Are Contracted

If a person is to become infected, he or she must first acquire the appropriate organism. There are several ways in which this can be done:

1. From already infected persons, obviously suffering from the disease (e.g. measles), or from infected persons *not* showing any signs of illness, as in the case of subclinical rubella infection.
2. From human carriers, either long term carriers such as those who carry the organism that causes typhoid fever or patients just recovered from infection but still harbouring the organism for a short time, as in poliomyelitis.
3. From infected animals, as is the case with rabies or psittacosis (parrot disease).
4. From the environment, e.g. food (food poisoning), water (typhoid fever, Legionnaire's disease).

Infection acquired from cases of infection

In some diseases infection always causes illness and there are no subclinical cases. This is true of measles so that a measles infection can be acquired only from another case of measles. In some other infections subclinical infection can occur, so that the patient will not know that he has been infected or that he has passed the infection on to a second person. This occurs in rubella (German measles) and poliomyelitis.

Infection acquired from carriers

People who continue to excrete the infecting organism for varying periods after they have recovered from the illness are known as carriers. There are two kinds.

After an infection by the virus of poliomyelitis (poliovirus) the patient continues to excrete the virus in his stools for about six weeks, by which time he will have recovered from the acute effects of the infection (if, indeed, any such effects were present; less than 1 per cent of those infected with the poliovirus have an illness). This period of excretion of the virus was a very important factor in the spread of poliomyelitis in the days before vaccination and still is in those countries where vaccination is not generally practised.

The other form of carrier is the one who goes on excreting the organism for long periods, even years. This may happen in hepatitis B infections and in typhoid fever and such carriers may be described as walking time-bombs.

Such a person was 'Typhoid Mary'. Her real name was Mary Mallon; by occupation she was a cook, operating mainly in New York. She moved from family to family, trailing cases of typhoid in her wake. In about 1907 her propensities were at last recognized and she was put into Riverside Hospital for Infectious Diseases where she remained for three years. During her stay there she worked as a laundress without causing any incident, so in 1910 she was released on condition that she remained a laundress, not a cook and that she reported every three months. Of course, she disappeared, working for five years in the kitchens of New York. There were many cases of typhoid fever in New York at that time, so that any cases that she might have caused were not investigated as to the source of the infection.

In 1915 there was a serious outbreak of typhoid fever in the Sloane Hospital for Women in New York, with twenty-five cases and two deaths. The staff jokingly referred to the cook there as 'Typhoid Mary' and she left at once—she really *was* 'Typhoid Mary'! The police then found her working in a kitchen on Long Island. After this it was necessary for her be kept in quarantine for life and she returned to Riverside Hospital and worked as a technician. In 1923 the city built her a cottage by the hospital, but in 1932 she suffered a stroke and died in November 1938. Her official score of cases was fifty-three with three deaths, but the real total must have been vastly greater and probably a great epidemic of 1,400 cases in Ithaca, New York in 1903 was due to her activities!

Animals and human infection

Animals are associated with infection in three different ways:

1. They may share infections with man.
2. They may carry infectious organisms purely mechanically.
3. They may be necessary for a certain phase of the development of the infecting organism.

An infection shared

Infections shared between animals and humans are known as 'zoonoses' and they occur commonly. For example, some infections that dogs may pass to humans are:

Rabies	Salmonella infection
Hydatid cyst	Fleas
Toxacara (a worm)	Hookworm
Ringworm	Tropical ulcers
Leptospirosis	Pasteurella infection

Some infections that can be contracted from cats are:

Ringworm	Leptospirosis
Cat-scratch fever	Salmonella infection
Toxoplasmosis	Fleas
Rabies	Pasteurella infection

Two good examples of zoonoses are rabies from dogs and bovine tuberculosis from cattle. The bovine tubercle bacillus is present in the milk of infected cows, so that, before the days of universal pasteurization of milk and tuberculin testing of dairy herds, this organism caused widespread illness in Britain. Because the infecting agent was swallowed rather than inhaled as with the human tubercle bacillus, the neck glands, bowel and bones were affected rather than the lungs so that fifty years ago scarred necks (following the surgical removal of tuberculous glands) were very common, as were 'spinal carriages'—virtual coffins on wheels occupied for long periods (usually terminated by death) by those whose spines had been eaten away by tuberculous abscesses.

In some cases there is free interchange of organisms between more than two species; cattle infected with a salmonella organism can infect the farm dog who in turn may infect the farmer's children.

Animals as mechanical carriers of infection

A variety of infections is passed on in this way. On a sheep farm where there is a high incidence of cysticercosis (the sheep/dog tapeworm) among the sheep, the pastures may be contaminated by the eggs of this worm. These may contaminate the fur of the sheepdog and be passed on to the shepherd when he pats or strokes the dog. After eating food that he may have contaminated by his hands the shepherd may develop a hydatid cyst.

The housefly has been shown to carry dysentery bacilli, because of its predilection for unpleasant substances. During the Second World War it was blamed extensively for the spread of this disease particularly in tropical stations and it was also accused of carrying the poliomyelitis virus, but it is not really known how important was the housefly's role in the spread of these infections.

Organisms that need to develop in another animal

In many cases an animal, almost always an arthropod, often a mosquito, provides a necessary environment for one part of the development of an organism, usually a single celled parasite. Malaria is a good example, in which the infection is contracted by the bite of a mosquito. The malarial parasite must go through several stages of development within the mosquito before it can infect man so that, immediately after it has bitten an infected patient, the mosquito is not yet infectious but only so after an interval of 8 to 35 days, when the malarial parasites within it will have matured.

Infection from the environment

A few hardy organisms survive happily in water and the soil and the tetanus bacillus is one of them. Another is the organism that causes, among other conditions, gas gangrene, an organism which is also carried harmlessly in the bowels of normal people (showing that the 'wrong' organism in the 'right' place may be harmless, but not when it gets into the 'wrong' place).

Cl. welchii cannot grow in the presence of oxygen, but damaged tissues are notoriously short of oxygen, so that infection with this organism can follow certain operations such as the pinning of the neck of the femur (hip) in old ladies. Because the hip is close to the bowel the organism frequently contaminates the skin. The operation of pinning causes some damage to the tissues and there is considerable bruising and bleeding locally. If *Cl. welchii* can just begin to multiply in the damaged tissue it can produce large volumes of gas and this has the effect of compressing the small blood vessels and reducing further the oxygen available to the tissues. (See Figure 2.1.)

Figure 2.1 Gas gangrene

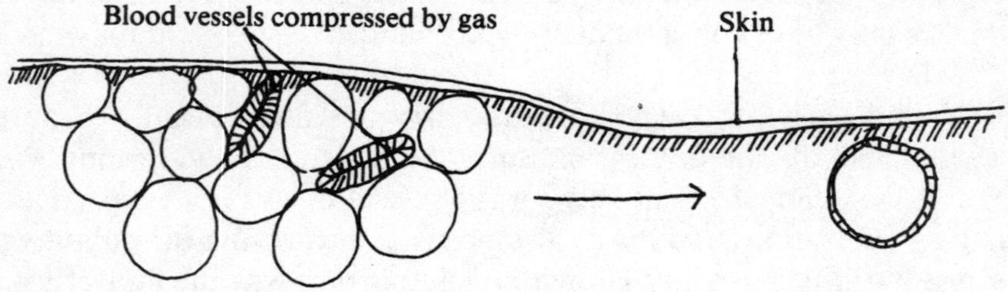

The gas gangrene bacilli produce gas, and it collects below the skin, generating enough pressure to compress the blood vessels; this prevents oxygen from reaching the tissues, allowing the organism to multiply and spread, which it could not do in the presence of oxygen.

As a result of this the organism can multiply further and so the infection can spread outward at an alarming rate, killing the tissue and producing a layer of gas below the skin that can be felt to crackle under the fingers. Such a condition may cause death within twelve hours but fortunately the infection can be prevented by providing the patient with a penicillin 'umbrella' during the period of the operation.

The organism can exist in dust and dirt so that, in a road traffic accident when the victim has a car bumper rammed into his person, as well as damaging the tissue this may also introduce a few gas gangrene organisms which can multiply in the damaged tissue if antibiotics are not given promptly. The same condition also occurred frequently in war conditions before the introduction of antibiotics.

Exits and entrances

In order to infect others the offending organism must leave the patient or carrier and enter a new victim. (See Figure 2.2.) The exit route from the patient or carrier and the entry route to the new victim depend on the sort of infection concerned.

Bowel infections

The infecting organisms pass out in the stools and may infect others by of one several routes. Among young children the standards of hygiene are low and the amount of bodily contact extreme, so that organisms that are usually spread by other well-defined ways are, among children, spread by direct contact. Thus dysentery may spread rapidly through a nursery school while the same infection in a responsible adult may not be passed on to a single person. One of the most important ways of preventing spread of bowel infection is by regular hand washing, especially after visiting the toilet.

Figure 2.2 The ins and outs of infection

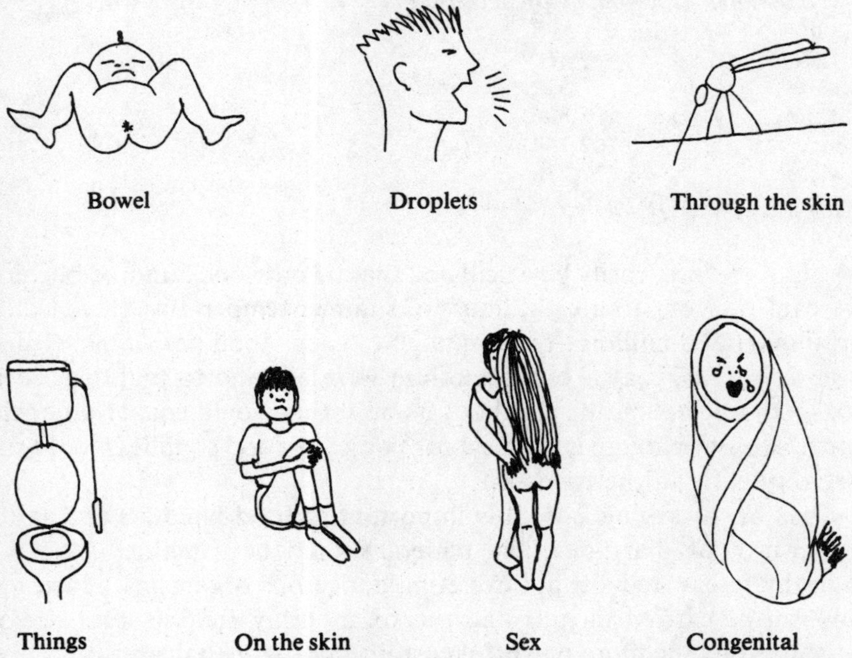

It is a well-known fact that toilet paper is not impervious to bacteria; long ago this was demonstrated to me by a professor of bacteriology. A stool on a plate was covered with a layer of toilet paper; I washed my hands well and then touched the 'clean' side of the paper and then placed my fingers on some solid medium. After incubation the latter showed an exact pattern of my fingerprints, worked in colonies of the organism present in the stools. If they had contained typhoid bacilli and I had not washed my hands after touching the toilet paper, I might well have developed typhoid fever.

In many instances there may be a further step in the path of infection.

My infected fingers, either as a result of the above infection or, more probably, following a more usual contact with contaminated toilet paper, might be used for preparing food.

Many foodstuffs are excellent media for the growth of bacteria – in fact, broth is still the most popular liquid medium, so that the dangerous organisms that might be transferred from my fingers to food would multiply rapidly in it.

In warm weather bacteria can divide every twenty minutes or so, and the growth of bacteria in terms of hours can be seen below:

Hours later	*Number of bacteria*
one	8
two	64
three	512
four	4,896
six	262,144
eight	16,777,216
twelve	over 8,000 million

It can, therefore, easily be calculated that, if only one hundred bacteria were introduced, after eight hours of summer temperature there would be about 1,500 million – quite enough to cause food poisoning. (It has been calculated that if one bacterium were allowed to multiply freely for forty-five hours, the weight of its offspring would equal that of the earth. However, there is no need for panic: its food supplies would run out very early in the process!)

Thus handwashing is doubly important in food handlers and, after any attack of diarrhoea, the patient should be examined bacteriologically to ensure he is not excreting dangerous organisms. However, this can be carried too far and the six monthly routine stool testing demanded by the more powerful customers of large bakeries is useless, as it only detects what is present at that time, and, in the absence of diarrhoea, there is unlikely to be anything worth finding.

Food poisoning at the seaside

Thirty or so years ago, Southend-on-Sea was the Mecca as far as club and pub outings were concerned. Frequently the participants complained about intestinal upsets following their visit, but it was rare that any specific organism was discovered. As the then Medical Officer of Health pointed out: 'They have a few drinks from the crate on the coach, then a few more on the seafront, a few plates of cockles or whelks, several more drinks and then several more on the way home. No wonder some of them suffer from "gastric upsets"!'

However on one occasion a pub outing came down to Southend, enjoyed the usual routine, but on the way home many of the participants became violently sick. When questioned about their intakes during the day it turned out that, in addition to the usual rich fare, they also partook of ham sandwiches prepared by the publican's wife. Some of the ham remained, and on examination it was found to be heavily contaminated with *Staphylococcus aureus*—a well-known cause of food poisoning. The publican's wife was questioned about its preparation and admitted cooking it a week before the outing. It could not have been contaminated, she pointed out, since between the cooking and the outing she had kept it under her bed!

Another route of bowel infection is through water supplies. In this country we are lucky enough to have a supply that is almost perfect, bacteriologically speaking, and this is true nearly all over Europe, although accidents can happen. In 1937, in Croydon there was a large outbreak of typhoid fever said to be caused by a workman working on a small reservoir who wished to pass water and used the reservoir rather than a toilet.

Cholera is a disease of refugees, when the poor people must use a single lake for washing, as a lavatory and for drinking purposes. It was truly said by Tom Lehrer that life is like a sewer—what you get out of it depends on what you put into it!

The part played by shellfish in spreading enteric infection will be discussed later.

Skin infections on the surface

These may be caused by contact with other infected skins—ringworm, for instance, may be contracted by children in this way. Only recently a rugby football club suspended its fixtures for a time because several of its forwards were suffering from impetigo, a disease transmissible by close skin contact in populations of children and of rugby forwards (I acquired it this way nearly fifty years ago) so that it is sometimes known as 'scrum pox'.

Some infections may be caused by both direct contact and through infected clothing. Scabies is such an infection. Nurses and dentists may acquire their first herpes infections on their fingers from contact with infected patients, while nurses and doctors may infect the operation wounds of patients if their hand washing precautions are not efficient.

Skin infection through the skin

This refers to infection acquired by skin puncture rather than simple infection of the surface. Until fairly recently diseases spread in this way occurred mainly in the tropics, where diseases such as malaria and yellow fever were acquired by the bites of mosquitoes. In recent years, however, the two diseases of hepatitis B and AIDS have been recognized. The former has spread rapidly, mainly through homosexual practices where there is a fair amount of abrasion to the parts employed so that the blood of one partner may get under the skin of the other; other modes of infection include sharing of syringes by drug addicts, ear piercing, acupuncture and tattooing. AIDS appears at present to be spread mainly by homosexual practices, by the sharing of syringes by drug addicts and, in the past, by blood transfusions and contaminated blood products (for haemophiliacs).

Sexually transmitted diseases

There is some overlap between these and those diseases caused by penetration of the skin, especially if we include homosexual intercourse, as both hepatitis B and AIDS can be acquired by both routes. Diseases like these used to be known as venereal diseases.

These infections will be dealt with in greater detail in another chapter; but it should be emphasized that the sexually transmitted infections are, in fact, transmitted by this method only because the organisms causing them are very delicate and fastidious and cannot withstand dry conditions or changes of temperature; thus they can be spread only when there is the very smallest gap for them to leap from one person to another. Thus transmission by lavatory seats is an explanation to be doubted even from the mouths of senior clerics!

Sexually transmitted infections are passed usually from man to woman (or vice versa) and they cause ulceration and discharge in the parts of both parties. However, anatomy encourages men to hold and inspect the affected part at every call of nature whereas, in women, the damage is hidden deep within (damage to the sword is more obvious than damage to the sheath!); in any case many women suffer, quite unnecessarily, from a continual innocent vaginal discharge.

Sexually transmitted diseases include gonorrhoea, syphilis, chlamydial infection, genital herpes, trichomonas infection, hepatitis B and AIDS.

Infection spread by coughing and sneezing

When she heard that as a doctor I would be dealing with tuberculous patients, my mother, a midwife, advised me: 'Don't get their breath, son.' This was good advice because many 'chest' diseases are acquired by inhaling organisms breathed or coughed out by infected patients. As well as the recognized 'chest' diseases, several infections usually thought of as 'general' infections, often with rashes, are acquired in this way.

Infection by a 'chest' organism, such as influenza, is acquired directly, that is, the organism is breathed into the lung where it acquires a foothold and multiplies, causing infection of the lung.

The organisms that cause the 'general' infections (e.g. measles and chickenpox) are breathed in the same way and they also infect the lung and multiply, but usually the effect on the lung is small, as it is merely the place where the organisms multiply before passing into the blood which carries them all over the body, involving many systems; the rash, for instance, indicates involvement of the skin. Other general diseases include rubella and glandular fever.

Coughs, colds, sore throats and scarlet fever are diseases of the respiratory tract spread by coughs and sneezes. When we cough or sneeze we expel droplets of mucus or saliva containing bacteria or viruses. These droplets have different fates according to their size. Droplets larger than 0.1 microns in diameter are on the heavy side and tend to fall downwards, on to the clothes or bedclothes, like soup from the spoon of a messy eater; subsequent shaking of the bedclothes will suspend the organisms present in the air, perhaps to be inhaled by others. The smaller droplets, less than 0.1 microns in size, float away and evaporate, leaving a tiny speck of dust containing organisms. These specks of dust are wafted on the breeze and may cause infection at a great distance away from the person from whom they originated. (See Figure 2.3.)

Congenital infections

Research into the causes of diseases with which babies are born suggest that there are two main forms:

1. Genetic diseases are due to defective or false information on the chromosomes of the child. The defect may have been present on a chromosome from the sperm or the egg (or both) or it may have arisen during the development of the embryo from a single cell.
2. Infectious diseases that affect the mother and are passed on to the

baby in the womb also cause handicaps in the child. Such infections include rubella, cytomegalovirus infection and toxoplasmosis.

Transplants, grafts and transfusions

As we shall see later, many viruses reside permanently in our bodies after the symptoms of infection have disappeared. Such viruses may be present in pieces of tissue (skin, cornea, kidneys and larger organs) or blood donated to a patient. Cytomgalovirus infection commonly affects those receiving kidney grafts and AIDS has been contracted through a corneal graft.

Figure 2.3 Droplet spread of infection

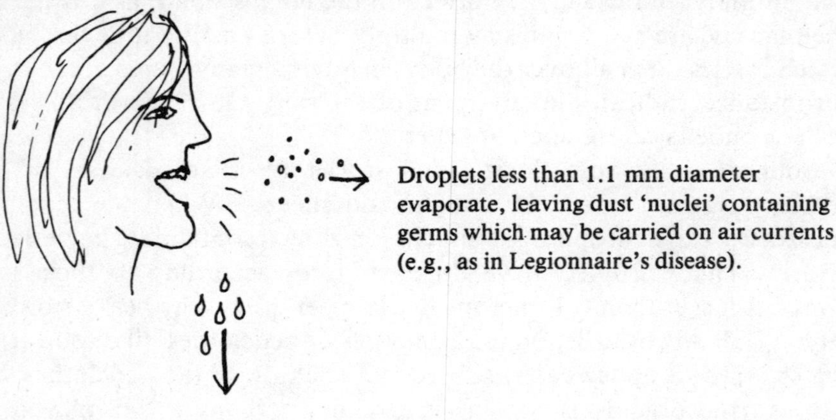

Another complication of transplant, described more fully in the next chapter, is that the body treats the new tissue as foreign matter and does its best to get rid of it—'graft rejection'. For this reason it is usual to destroy medically the immunity of transplant patients to prevent graft rejection; unfortunately, this loss of immunity prevents the patient from rejecting any little non-optional extras in the form of viruses resident in the graft, so that many develop a severe infection after, for instance, a kidney transplant.

A patient undergoing transplant surgery often needs a blood transfusion and any organism latent in the transfused blood may cause severe illness in the patient.

Spread by fomites

Fomites is the plural of the Latin 'fomes', meaning 'tinder', that is, something that may be handled by many people in a short period of time (in the way that, in the days when many more people smoked, it might have been possible to catch an infection by passing a cigarette lighter from hand to hand). The term is now applied to any inanimate object that might carry infectious organisms. This could be a pencil sucked by several schoolchildren or a complicated artificial respiration machine.

In hospitals much attention has to be paid to the various 'scopes' used by doctors to peer into a patient's various orifices because these instruments have been known to carry infection from patient to patient. Shared syringes and needles have been mentioned and shared razors might spread hepatitis type B as well as HIV infection that can cause AIDS.

Epidemics

An epidemic is 'something put upon the people' (in the Biblical sense) – a sudden increase of the incidence of a disease in a community. If there is a worldwide increase then it is known as a pandemic. This is usually due to the emergence of a new organism or a strain quite different from previous strains. When a disease is always present in a given community, but on a small scale, it is said to be endemic. An 'epidemic' among animals is, strictly speaking, an epizootic. Diseases spread from animals to man are known as zoonoses.

Epidemics need special conditions to occur, generally speaking, a large proportion of susceptible (i.e. not immune) people in the population and a large amount of the infecting agent in the environment.

Epidemics and immunity

Immediately after an epidemic most of the population will have been infected, either recently or earlier. Thus most of the population will be immune and few infections will occur although the organism will be still present in the small number of cases still occurring (the infection has become endemic). As time goes by more children are born and these will eventually provide a large enough group of susceptible persons for an epidemic to occur again. In the past epidemics of whooping cough and measles have occurred every five years or so but today, the picture is less clearcut because of vaccination (to such an extent that if the vaccination had been sufficiently vigorously carried out epidemics of these preventable diseases would no longer occur).

Another factor in the emergence of epidemics is the availability of the infecting organism. In most infections the source is other patients, but as the number of susceptibles becomes smaller, the number of infecting sources becomes smaller and it becomes less likely that one of the few remaining susceptibles will come in contact with one of the few remaining cases. When the local standards of hygiene are low and especially when, at the same time, the water supply is the source of infection there is a much greater opportunity for the remaining susceptibles to be infected from the water – a large and constant source of infection. This is the situation that occurs when a refugee camp is attacked by cholera and it may also occur in military situations where victory rather than hygiene is the immediate goal.

We should also remember the fact that during wars the incidence of sexually transmitted diseases may reach epidemic proportion. In the past, when the main weapon against syphilis was mercury ointment, it used to be said that where Mars was you would discover Venus and Mercury would not be far away. Penicillin has ruined that epigram!

THREE

Immunity: Avoiding Infection

The word immunity comes from the Latin *im* (not) and *munus* (to serve). During Roman times people who had served the state in some special way were exempted from military duty or from taxes—they were said to be 'immune' from these impositions. The meaning of the word has been extended to include freedom from infection or, rather, freedom from contracting infection. Although we talk of 'immunity' in the singular, the word denotes a rich and complex variety of cells and series of reactions that act together to prevent infection.

There are two separate aspects of immunity: one being general and directed against *all* infecting agents, while the other is special or specific and depends on the body having knowledge of a particular infecting organism in the past and remembering it in the future—thus this sort of immunity depends on previous infection or vaccination. It is as if there were two sorts of crime prevention officer, one that acts immediately when he sees the law broken and a second who has the ability to recognize known criminals and to act accordingly.

Nonspecific or general immunity

There are many ways by which the body discourages invasion by infecting organisms. The easiest of these to understand is how the skin provides a wall which covers the whole of the body. This is a fairly thick mechanical barrier armed with various glands that produce sweat and similar substances which are antibacterial. When the skin is breached infection can readily occur and this is seen quite often following surgical operations, after the surgeon has made a hole in the skin. Again, infection is one of the serious complications of extensive burns that have destroyed the skin, when organisms that normally cause little harm on the surface of the body or within the bowel are able to grow in wounds and cause severe infection.

This is one of the basic facts of infection: *that some organisms may be quite harmless when in their usual habitats, e.g. on the intact skin or within the bowel, but when they find themselves in less rugged areas of the body, as in wounds, on the surface of the brain, in joints or in the kidney, they are able to cause severe infection and often death.*

Wounds, then, are very susceptible sites and the largest wound commonly encountered is that left behind in the womb after delivery of the baby and before the womb contracts down to its normal non-pregnant size. In the past many deaths have followed infection of this area, often by the hands of the midwife or doctor.

In 1846, long before Pasteur had discovered bacteria, a Dr Semmelweiss was appointed as Director of the Obstetric Department of the General Hospital in Vienna, which was then the biggest maternity hospital in the world. The hospital was divided into two parts or clinics; Clinic 1 consisted of five wards on which doctors and medical students were taught and Clinic 2 consisted of five wards on which midwives were taught. The mortality for mothers on Clinic 2 was a massive 6 per cent but that for Clinic 1 was even greater at 18 per cent. It must be remembered that these were normal maternity cases—until they entered this hospital!

Austria was, and still is, a religious country and last rites were administered to all mothers about to die. Unfortunately the geography of the wards was such that the chapel was next to Clinic 2 so that the robed and chanting priests had to pass through all five wards of Clinic 2 before reaching their dying charges in Clinic 1. Thus the morale was as low as the mortality rate was high in this hospital.

At this time pathologists had not yet appeared on the medical scene so that doctors and students used to carry out post-mortem examinations for themselves. These examinations would usually be performed in the early morning before the ward round and on these rounds the doctors and students would normally carry out internal examinations on the unfortunate women. As they expected to get their hands dirty anyway they did not usually trouble to wash before doing this, intending to have a good wash before finishing for lunch.

In 1847 a colleague of Dr Semmelweiss cut himself while carrying out a post-mortem, developed blood poisoning and died. At the post-mortem examination Dr Semmelweiss was struck by the resemblance between the post-mortem appearance of his unfortunate colleague and that seen in the post-mortem examination of those women who had died. He rightly surmised that the doctors and students might be carrying something from the post-mortem room to the wards on their hands. He decreed that all doctors and students should henceforward wash their hands in a solution of chloride of lime before examining patients. When this was done the mortality rate in Clinic 1 fell from 18 per cent to 1 per cent, while in clinic 2 it fell from 6 per cent to 1 per cent.

Unfortunately, Semmelweiss's discovery was not acceptable to the bigoted European medical world of that time and he had not the character to stand up to his critics. He had to be admitted to a mental hospital where, ironically, he died after a few weeks from blood poisoning caused by a cut he made to his hand during his final operation before incarceration.

Another body mechanism that helps to avoid infection is found in the lungs. As we saw earlier, many infectious agents are inhaled and begin to multiply in the lungs (the air passages to be precise). These passages are lined with cells carrying little hairlike processes called 'cilia' that flick in one direction, rather like the spectators at a Mexican football match. There are also a large number of minute glands that produce a sticky substance called mucus. Organisms settling on the surface of the air passages become entangled in the mucus and made up into a tiny parcels which are flicked upwards by the little hairs. When they reach the larynx, the patient becomes aware of them and coughs them up into the mouth where they are either swallowed—and dealt with by the acid in the stomach—or spat out. (See Figure 3.1.)

The stomach acid is also important in that it kills many, but not all, of the infectious organisms that enter the body by that route. People who lack stomach acid are more likely to develop bowel infections than those with it and monkeys given poliovirus after a meal, which neutralizes the acid, are more likely to develop poliomyelitis than those that receive it on an empty stomach.

Specific immunity

One of the most remarkable characteristics of the higher animals is the ability of their bodies to remember details of organisms that have previously infected them, to produce means of fighting these organisms and then being able to recognize them and mobilize these special forces against them when a second infection occurs.

Figure 3.1 Protection of the air passages of the lungs

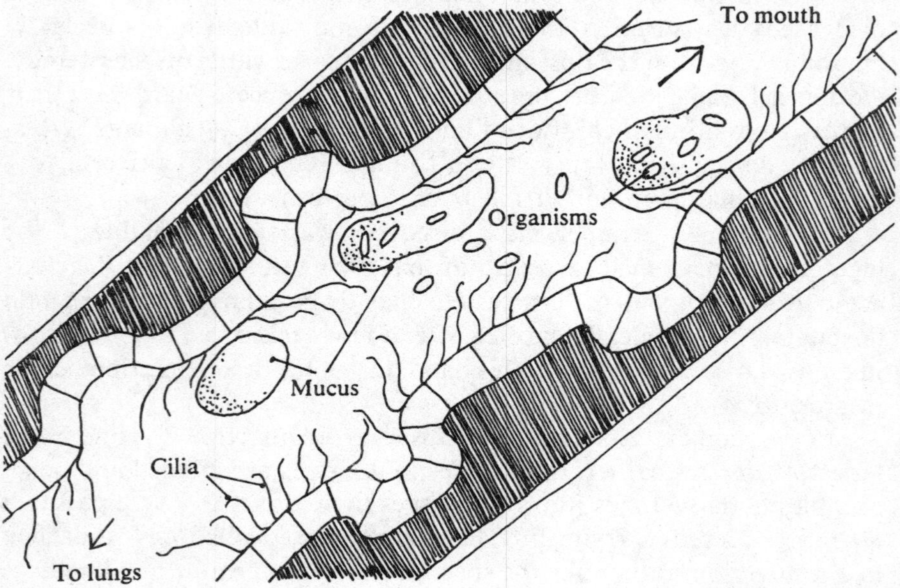

The mucus that contains bacteria is rolled up into little balls and flicked up towards the mouth.

Substances that are able to cause an 'immune reaction' are called 'antigens' and have two important qualities:

1. They have large molecules, being usually proteins or large carbohydrate molecules – the 'carrier'.
2. Each different sort of antigen carries on its surface a specific chemical pattern – the 'hapten'.

The antigen can be likened to a key; the hapten is specific and resembles the 'blade' of the key. The carrier resembles the handle, which if it is not large enough means that the key cannot be used.

Antigens

The antigens that are important in infection consist of infectious organisms or parts of them, although pollen, dust and other substances can act as antigens in causing allergic reactions. Also, artificial antigens can be made in the laboratory by attaching relatively simple chemical groups to proteins.

The immune response

This is the name given to those changes that occur in the body in response to an antigen and which are mainly directed towards preventing infection by the same organism in the future. The general mode of action is as follows:

1. Antigen (usually an infecting organism or part of it) stimulates certain white cells in the blood or lymph glands to multiply; these cells produce:
   a. Antibody-producing cells.
   b. 'Anti-infector' cells.
   c. Memory cells.
2. These cells have very little effect on the current infection as they are too few and too late.
3. If the patient recovers from the first infection he is left with memory cells in his blood and lymph glands. If he becomes infected by the same organism again, the 'memory cells' will multiply rapidly giving rise to many antigen-producing cells and anti-infector cells.
4. The antibody-producing cells produce antibody in realistic amounts and this tends to abort the infection.
5. The anti-infector cells act in various ways:
   a. Some help the antigen-producing cells to produce more antigen—these are the T-helper cells.
   b. Others attack organisms directly.
   c. They train large cells—macrophages—to seek out and destroy the offending organisms.
   d. They control the movements of other white cells to and from the site of infection. (See Figure 3.2.)

Antibody

Antibodies are a group of substances that appear in the blood as a result of stimulation by antigen and they belong to a group of proteins known as 'immunoglobulins'. Precisely how they deal with invading organisms is not fully understood, but in the laboratory they tend to bind together bacteria in a process called 'agglutination'; it is as if a gang of bank robbers were bound together with sticky tape, which would seriously hamper their activities. (See Figure 3.3.) Another mechanism is by

Figure 3.2 Infection and immunity

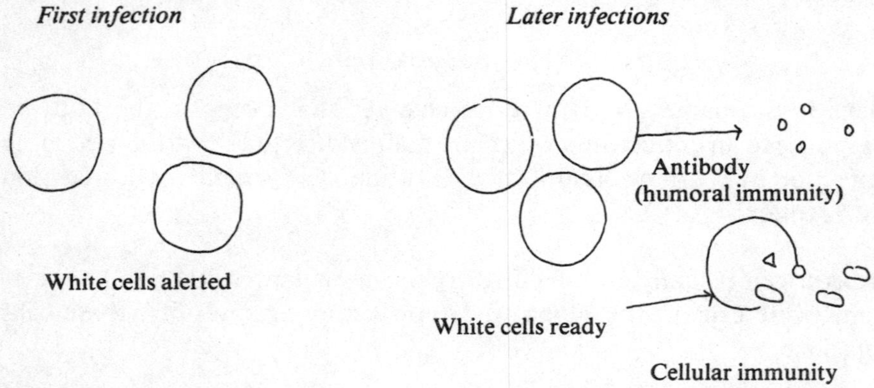

cooperating with a substance called 'complement', present in the blood; together the two substances pierce holes in foreign cells (especially the red ones) and allow the contents to leak out. The immunity produced by antibody is known as 'humoral' immunity as opposed to 'cellular' immunity when cells attack invaders directly.

Figure 3.3 Antibody causes agglutination

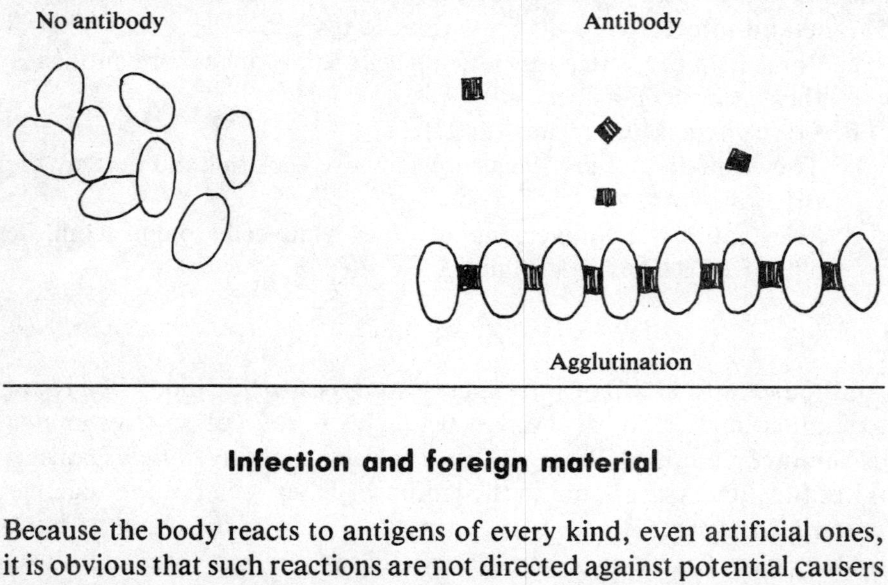

Infection and foreign material

Because the body reacts to antigens of every kind, even artificial ones, it is obvious that such reactions are not directed against potential causers of harm as such but towards all foreign substances that may be antigenic and which find themselves within the body. Thus the body is not able to distinguish between *harmful* agents such as bacteria and potentially *helpful* substances such as transfused blood of a different blood group or a transplanted heart or kidney.

Immune tolerance

It is not known precisely what mechanism prevents the body from mounting immune responses to its own tissues. However, certain religious orders have boasted that, if given the child during his formative years, he will be theirs for life; ideas that he might consider ridiculous if encountered later in life when his critical faculties had developed may be tolerated for life if first encountered in early childhood.

This phenomenon has its parallel in immunity; if an antigen is injected into a newborn animal before its immune mechanism has developed completely, no antibody will be produced towards that antigen. If, when the animal becomes mature, the same antigen is injected, still no antibody is produced. The body has come to regard the foreign antigen as being truly of itself. This process is known as 'immune tolerance'.

Immunity and graft rejection

From what has been written so far, it will be obvious that a graft derived from another individual will probably be regarded as foreign and rejected. The rejection is mainly caused by the action of cells (cellular immunity), but a transplant of skin from another part of the anatomy of the same individual will 'take'. Related people tend to have a similar antigenic make-up so that an antigenic match between identical twins is practically certain, between a parent and child once in two occasions, between brother/sister about once in four occasions and for complete strangers only once in many hundreds of thousands.

For this reason, whenever possible, transplants are taken from close relatives of the patient—for instance a kidney from a twin. In the case of heart transplant this is, of course, impossible, as it is not likely that twin will die at the right time! After the transplant of an organ from a stranger, it is necessary to destroy, temporarily, the patient's immunity. This can be done using drugs and antisera but during the course of this procedure the patient becomes very vulnerable to all sorts of infectious agents—he suffers from 'medically induced AIDS'. During this period of immunosuppression the patient must be nursed in an environment that is as germ-free as is humanly possible and treated with antibiotics at the first sign of infection. Fortunately, after a while, when the graft or transplant has taken, the patient's immunity slowly returns.

Making use of immunity

If an attack of infection usually renders a person immune to further attacks, then why not seek ways of giving people mild or even completely symptom-free attacks of the important infectious diseases so as to confer immunity to these diseases upon them? This idea has been developed over a long period, giving rise to the practice of vaccination as used today.

The prevention of smallpox

The prevention of smallpox by giving the patient a mild attack of the disease was investigated by the Chinese in the Middle Ages, when they dried smallpox crusts and ground them into snuff. This was called 'Heavenly Flowers' and when sniffed it gave a vaccinia 'take' inside the nose, which must have been very painful. Often the disease became generalized and also spread to other persons, sometimes with fatal results. Lady Mary Wortley Montagu, a formidable English lady explorer of the eighteenth century, brought back the method of 'variolation' for this purpose. Material from a 'spot' on a mild case of smallpox was injected into the skin of the subject. The same disadvantages followed this practice as followed the use of 'Heavenly Flowers'; about one patient in 300 died.

Dr Edward Jenner, a family doctor in Gloucestershire, heard, as a young man, that anyone who had had cowpox did not take smallpox. It was not until twenty-five years later that he had time to follow up this theory. He began by using his son as a guinea-pig and inoculated him, in the first case, with swinepox material at the age of ten months and then with infectious smallpox material on five or six occasions, failing each time to cause the disease. Nothing if not thorough, Jenner repeated the smallpox injections when the boy was two and again a year later. Although the boy did not get smallpox he developed skin infections because of the presence of other infectious organisms in the impure material used. Jenner's biographer said later of the boy: 'He had always been delicate in health and, moreover, had a rather defective understanding.' This seems hardly surprising.

In 1796 a milkmaid, Sarah Neames, developed cowpox – small

blisters on the fingers through infection from the cow's teats. In May of that year James Phipps, age eight, was inoculated by Jenner with material from Sarah's wrist and developed a small blister at the site of inoculation. Six weeks later Jenner injected him with smallpox material but he did not develop the disease. During the next twenty years Jenner tested Phipps at least twenty times with infectious smallpox material. Phipps was lucky and survived.

It was possible to obtain children from the local workhouse in those days and Jenner used at least two such boys for research. John Baker, age five, was injected with material from a patient with possible horse-pox and William Summers, also five, with matter from an infected cow teat. Baker was not tested with smallpox material because, in Jenner's words; 'The boy was rendered unfit for inoculation from having felt the effects of a contagious fever in the workhouse soon after the experiment was made'. Baker's ulcer spread and he died a few days later, possibly from erysipelas. Jenner was, of course, not aware of the multiplicity of infectious organisms that might be found on animals and today his behaviour would be regarded as criminally reckless.

The first report by Jenner on the use of cowpox to prevent smallpox was rejected but eventually he gained support from the medical profession after a great deal of sometimes bitter criticism. Because the material used was obtained from a cow, the procedure was called vaccination (Latin *vaccus*, a cow). When, later, Pasteur introduced immunization against rabies he called the procedure vaccination again, rather in honour of Jenner than in biological accuracy. The material originally used by Jenner for vaccination came, no doubt, from cowpox. Later on there was some doubt and it is likely that the material used in recent years for smallpox eradication and called vaccinia was really a strain of the smallpox virus that had lost its power to cause general infection through being grown in calves over many years.

The use of smallpox vaccine was made compulsory in Great Britain in 1853 and remained so until 1971.

Although Jenner received most of the honours when it was finally established that vaccination against smallpox was effective—and it is directly through his work that there has not been a case of smallpox in the world since the last occurred in Somalia on 26 October 1977—he was not the first to vaccinate. Priority goes to a Dorset farmer, Benjamin Jesty, who vaccinated his wife and two young children with matter from a sore on a cow's udder. Although smallpox was widespread in his county at the time, his family did not contract it. This occurred twenty-two years before Jenner first vaccinated and, although Jesty at first was very unpopular locally, he was 'adopted' by the 'Vaccine Pock Institute' of London, which was a rival of the institute set up by Jenner, leading to the usual bitter controversy that new medical procedures seem to attract.

The work of Louis Pasteur

Little more was done in the field of preventing infectious diseases by vaccination until the appearance of Louis Pasteur (1822–95). His interest was stimulated in an unusual way. He had already established that many infections were caused by minute living organisms – bacteria. He had showed that similar organisms were universally present in the air and on surfaces. He showed that there were many different types, especially in his work on beer.

When the French beer industry was about to be ruined because all the beer it produced was 'going off', Pasteur looked at the deposit from beer though his microscope and saw that in the good beer there was a deposit of yeast cells, while in the bad beer there was a deposit of bacteria; he also saw that the deposits were quite different in appearance. He introduced the process of pasteurization, heating the beer to about 60°C to kill the bacteria and then adding some yeast from a good fermentation; it is interesting to find that the process of pasteurization was used on beer before being applied to milk!

However, Pasteur was also interested in the effects on fowls of the organisms of 'Fowl Cholera'. He found that when injected with a small part of a culture of this organism chickens developed serious diarrhoea and died rapidly. On one occasion he began some new work on this subject and asked his assistant for a culture of the appropriate organism. His assistant had recently returned from holiday and had not had time to produce a fresh culture, so he produced one that had been made some weeks before. When the chickens were injected with this culture, some became slightly ill but all recovered quickly. Pasteur ordered a fresh culture to be made and he injected this into the birds and was surprised when they refused to die. Pasteur then reasoned that the old culture had been able to produce immunity in the chickens but not able to harm them; he then developed the concept that it was possible to alter organisms so that they would do this to order.

The first disease Pasteur tackled was anthrax, a serious disease of farm animals in those days. He showed that if anthrax bacilli were grown at a temperature a few degrees higher than that they seemed to like best, they were capable of infecting and immunizing but not of causing illness. Like Jenner, he received much criticism, but he was able to deal with it.

He organized a public experiment at a farm in a village near Melun in France. On 5 May 1881, 24 sheep, 1 goat and 6 cows were injected with six drops of the weakened anthrax culture. Twelve days later these animals, together with a further 24 sheep, 1 goat and 4 cows, were injected with fully active anthrax bacilli. Pasteur predicted that by 5 June at the latest the result of the experiment would be known. By 2 June all the vaccinated sheep were well, 21 control sheep and the goat had died, 2 control sheep died before the eyes of the spectators and the last 2 were dead by the end of the day. This experiment was carried out under almost fairground conditions (beautifully depicted in the 1936 film *The Story of Louis Pasteur*), the publicity was enormous and the scientific basis of vaccination had been established.

The next disease Pasteur dealt with was rabies—as we shall see this is a disease of dogs and wolves in Europe and, towards the end of the last century, shepherds appeared to be at great risk from bites by wolves. In dogs it causes illness just as it does in humans and is always fatal within fourteen days, so that when there is some risk that a bite is from a rabid dog, the latter must be kept confined for fourteen days and, if it does not become ill and die during this period, then it did not carry the rabies virus. Pasteur inherited relatively little information about rabies, although he knew:

It was transmitted through the saliva of a mad animal.
It was passed on through bites.
The incubation period varied from a few days to several months.

Pasteur showed that rabbits could be infected by rabies virus and that the spinal cords of such rabbits carried the virus and were infectious for other rabbits and dogs. If the infected rabbit's spinal cord was allowed to dry in air, after fourteen days it no longer caused illness in dogs; a dog could be injected with some '14-day' cord, then some '13-day' cord and so on until it was receiving fresh cord that killed other, uninoculated dogs. Hence the dog receiving dried cord had been made immune to the disease.

Did this method work for humans? Pasteur was not Jenner and was thus reluctant to use this new substance on humans despite an offer from the Emperor of Mexico to keep him supplied with condemned prisoners. However, on 6 July 1885, a nine-year-old boy from Alsace, Joseph Meister, was brought by his mother to Pasteur. The boy had been bitten two days before by a rabid dog and the local doctor, who knew of Pasteur's work, had sent the boy directly to him. Pasteur knew that the boy would certainly die if not treated, so, after consultation with his colleagues he injected the boy with a drop of extract from a 14-day spinal cord, using the recently invented hypodermic syringe. The course of the treatment lasted ten days and the last dose was from a cord dried for one day only and capable of killing rabbits in seven days. The boy's wound healed and he did not develop rabies. He became devoted to the cause of Pasteur and eventually became caretaker of the Pasteur Institute in Paris; sadly, he killed himself when the Germans marched into Paris in 1940.

Pasteur's contributions to the study of infections were considerable and his achievements included the following.

He showed that fermentation was caused by microbes.
He showed that these microbes were offspring of other microbes and did not just appear from nowhere.
He 'pasteurized' beer.
He expanded Jenner's work on vaccination through fowl cholera, anthrax and rabies.

Other Vaccines

Towards the end of the last century most of the different bacteria causing infections were discovered and during the first twenty or so years of this century many of the vaccines used today were developed – these will be discussed with the appropriate infections. However, at that time, viruses could not be grown in the laboratory so that it was not until after 1946, when methods of growing viruses in tissue culture were discovered, that vaccines could be prepared against infections like measles and rubella.

Antisera

Vaccination works by stimulating the body to produce antibodies and other substances which will prevent future infection by the organism present in the vaccine. It is, of course, specific: whooping cough vaccine will protect against whooping cough only and not against diphtheria or other infectious organisms. (See Figure 3.4.) (Our fathers and mothers often spoke about having been 'vaccinated', referring to smallpox vaccination, the only available vaccine in their days.)

Because there is sometimes a degree of urgency in producing immunity and the body works fairly slowly in producing antibody, we can,

Figure 3.4 Vaccination is specific

Vaccine	*Infection*	*Result*
Whooping cough	Whooping cough	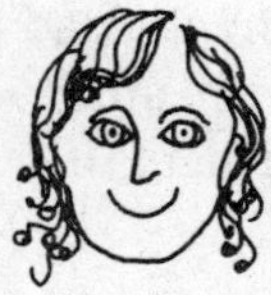
Tetanus	Tetanus	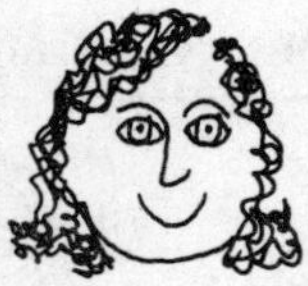
Whooping cough	Tetanus	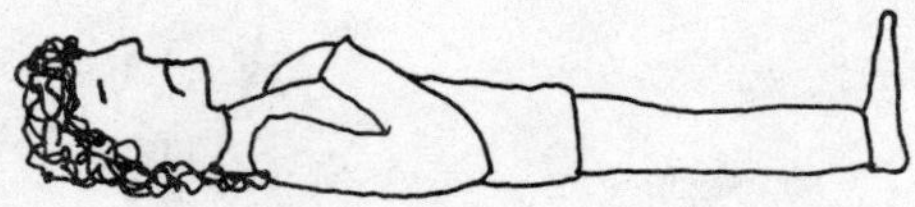

for instance in the case of a delicate child exposed to measles, offer the patient some ready-made antibody which will begin to work immediately on injection. (See Figure 3.5.)

These antisera may be obtained from two different sources—originally they were obtained by vaccinating horses with, for instance, diphtheria toxin. The horse produced antibody after a while, then it was bled and the blood serum used to treat children infected with the diphtheria bacillus. Unfortunately, horse serum contains horse protein which will produce antibodies in the patient who receives it; if this patient is given a second dose sometime later, he risks a serious reaction or possibly death.

Some years ago a fellow consultant brought his wife to me. While inspecting a house, she had stepped on a nail; although the risk of tetanus was slight, my colleague wanted his wife to be given tetanus antiserum. However, he was apprehensive about this. Many years ago his wife's sister had had the same experience and her father, a family doctor, had given her a full dose of antiserum, and she, being highly allergic, had died within five minutes. It is not surprising that I had all the apparatus for resuscitation at hand when I made the injection, but, fortunately, she did not turn a hair.

The other source of antiserum is from humans with a high level of it in their blood. Most normal people will have been infected by measles, chickenpox and hepatitis A during their lifetime, so that if the serum from blood, given for transfusion purposes but not used, is pooled, it is bound to have a reasonable level of antibodies to these infections. Thus people travelling abroad to unhygenic places may be given a dose of pooled normal serum antibody (often called 'gamma globulin') to prevent them acquiring hepatitis A.

Figure 3.5 Vaccines versus antisera

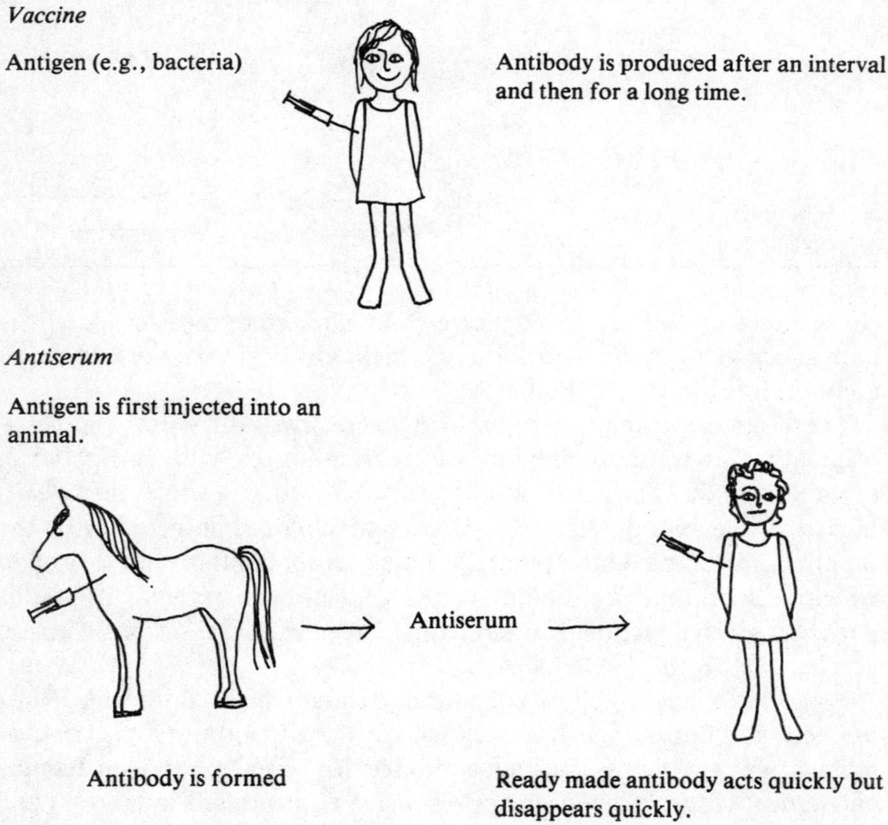

Because the body itself is not 'topping up' this extraneous antibody continuously, it will be gradually broken down and not replaced, but will remain active long enough to protect the patient for about three months.

Diseases of immunity

The immune mechanisms can go wrong:

1. Deficient immunity – either congenital or acquired. Acquired type includes AIDS and treatment to prevent graft rejection.
2. Inability to distinguish between the helpful and harmful.
3. Over-reaction to harmless antigen, e.g. asthma.
4. Autoimmunity – antibodies are formed that will destroy the patient's own tissues.

The immune mechanisms may be likened to a guard dog who usually can be relied upon but who occasionally slips up.

1. *Some guard dogs are not up to the job and sleep all the time.*
This is analagous with the condition of deficient immunity (the patient is 'immunodeficient') when the immune processes do not protect against infection. This condition may be present at birth or acquired later in life. Babies with severe immunodeficiency may die before diagnosis (immunodeficiency may be one cause of 'cot death'). Fortunately, during pregnancy, some of the mother's antibodies enter the baby's bloodstream – this provides him with antibody to several important infectious organisms.

These antibodies last for about six months, after which time the baby will normally be making his own antibody. But babies are variable and some will be 'late starters' and not produce antibody for up to eighteen months; it is quite impossible to distinguish between these late starters and those babies who never will produce antibody. Both these groups of babies will need to be given antibody from normal people for some time, the late starter until he eventually begins to make his own antibody and the non-starter for life.

Occasionally the immune system breaks down later in life, sometimes following exposure to toxic substances and sometimes during the course of illness, such as leukaemia or Hodgkin's Disease. Today a more dramatic cause of failure of the immune system has emerged in the form of AIDS (Acquired Immune Deficiency Syndrome), which is caused by a virus. In addition, as we have seen, it is necessary occasionally to destroy the immune system to prevent graft rejection.

2. *The guard dog cannot distinguish between a burglar and rich Uncle Percy from Australia, as he does not know either of them.*
The body cannot distinguish between *helpful* and *harmful* foreign sub-

stances and is stupid enough to reject a new heart in the same way as it rejects harmful bacteria and viruses.

3. *Some guard dogs over-react and bark hysterically at everybody and sometimes at nothing at all.*
The immunological equivalent is allergy and hypersensitivity, when the body over-reacts to harmless substances like dust or pollen.

A serious form of over-reaction which might fall into either of the above two categories is 'Rhesus Sensitivity' in pregnancy. Rhesus factors are simply chemical substances on the surface of red cells. If a woman who does not have these factors (i.e. is rhesus negative) becomes pregnant with a baby that does have these substances (rhesus positive), then, when the baby is born, a few drops of the baby's blood may enter the mother's circulation. As she does not posses the rhesus factors, there is every possibility of the mother making antibodies to the rhesus factors introduced into her circulation. As the 'current' baby has already been born, he will not be harmed, but if a subsequent pregnancy involves a baby that is again rhesus positive, the mother's rhesus antibody will attack the new baby's red cells, destroying them. When this occurs the only cure is a complete exchange transfusion at (or before) birth. (See Figure 3.6.)

Figure 3.6 Rhesus sensitivity – baby is Rh positive, but mother is Rh negative

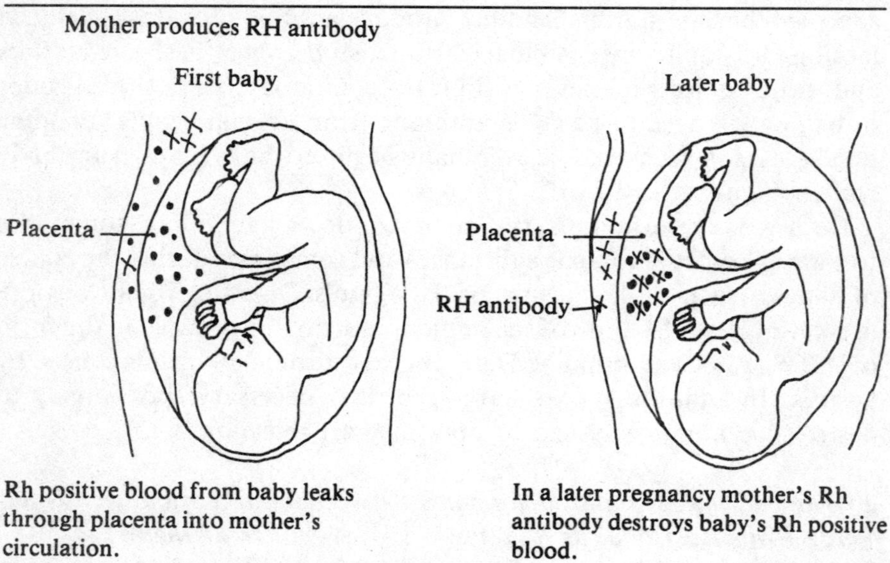

Rh positive blood from baby leaks through placenta into mother's circulation.

In a later pregnancy mother's Rh antibody destroys baby's Rh positive blood.

If it is known that a rhesus negative mother is carrying a rhesus positive baby for the first time, the mother can be prevented from producing rhesus antibody by the injection of a small amount of ready-made rhesus antibody immediately after the baby's birth; this will 'mop up' any rhesus positive cells from the baby that may have wandered into the mothers circulation. (See Figure 3.7.)

Figure 3.7 Preventing rhesus sensitivity by injecting rhesus antibody

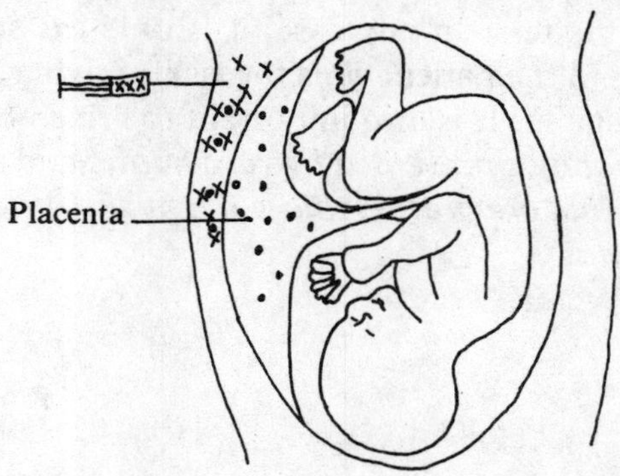

If Rhesus antibody is injected into the mother soon after delivery of the first (rhesus positive) baby, it 'mops up' any rhesus positive cells that may have leaked across the placenta.

4. *Some guard dogs turn on their masters and savage them.*
As we have seen, it is a matter of speculation as to why we do not produce antibody to our own tissues. The old scientists invoked a principle of 'Horror autotoxicus'—a fear of self-poisoning (this was the old trick of giving a name to a gap in our knowledge and pretending that it explained the matter).

However, we know now that, especially in later life, we do produce antibodies towards our own tissues and that more and more diseases whose causes could not be formerly explained are due, completely or in part, to our own antibody eroding our own tissues. Some people develop antibody to their own thyroid tissues and suffer from thyroid deficiency; rheumatoid arthritis—not to be confused with acute rheumatic fever—is a severe crippling disease caused by the body producing antibody to the membranes of the joints. This damages the joint surfaces and accounts for the severe pain and deformity that occurs in this disease. Some auto-immune conditions are as follows:

Thyroid disease	Male infertility
Pernicious anaemia	Rheumatoid arthritis
Some other anaemias	Ulcerative colitis

Postcript

This brief and incomplete account of immunity has shown that the body has modified its method of dealing with foreign substances into a method of preventing infection. It is not a fool-proof system, and, as the body is foolish, it cannot distinguish between benign and malignant foreign matters. In any case, it is only the second infection that is prevented and the patient runs the risk of dying from the first unless suitably vaccinated. It is also important to remember that *not all infectious diseases can be prevented by vaccination* and also that *vaccination against those that are preventable is not available to the majority of the earth's inhabitants*.

FOUR

Infection During Pregnancy

On the whole pregnancy is a time when a woman feels more healthy than ever before; however some infectious conditions can occur in pregnancy that may cause damage to the unborn child. Although this does not happen often it is important to take the necessary steps to prevent such infections.

Different infections are important at different stages of pregnancy and immediately afterwards:

1. *Early pregnancy*
   Rubella
   Cytomegalovirus infection
   Toxoplasmosis
   Listeriosis
2. *Late pregnancy*
   Chickenpox
   Vaccinia
   Hepatitis B
   Listeriosis
3. *During birth*
   Chlamydia
   Chickenpox
   Gonococci
   Herpes simplex
   Hepatitis B
   Listeriosis
4. *Neonatal period*
   Streptococci

Hepatitis B
Chickenpox
Cytomegalovirus infection
Rotavirus
Listeriosis

Rubella

Rubella is a mild disease that affects most people at some time: in females who are not pregnant and in males it causes only a temperature, enlarged lymph glands, a rash and, especially in adults, painful joints.

Rubella during pregnancy

In 1941 Norman Gregg, an Australian eye surgeon, dealt with a large number of cases of congenital cataracts—that is, babies with scars on the lens of the eye. These scars caused either total or partial blindness and some of the babies also had defective hearts. There had been an epidemic of rubella earlier that year and of seventy-eight infants with cataracts sixty-eight of the mothers had suffered from rubella during pregnancy. Gregg immediately decided that the cataracts were caused by rubella infection in the uterus. However, he had great difficulty in convincing the medical world that this was so. However, after about six years a sufficient number of careful surveys had been carried out to prove that rubella was, indeed, a frequent cause of handicaps in babies.

The importance of the stage pregnancy has reached when infection by rubella occurs is shown in the following:

Time of infection	*Percentage of babies affected*
Just before conception and up to 8 weeks	60–70
8–12 weeks	20–25
12–28 weeks	5–18

As can be seen, rubella does the greatest harm if infection occurs during the first three months of pregnancy and also if it occurs in the month before conception. Damage occasionally follows infection after the fourth month of pregnancy, but less frequently than after earlier infection.

As we have seen viruses often invade cells, multiply in them and then destroy them. In the developing baby the different organs all start as single cells of the appropriate kind which multiply so that, in their early stages, organs consist of a few cells only. At this time the destruction of a single cell will cause serious damage; if, on the other hand, the mature organ, consisting of millions of cells is attacked, it will be little damaged by the destruction of a few cells; it is the developing organ that is at risk. The lens of the eye, the inner ear and the heart all possess cells for which the rubella virus has an affinity and infection of these cells early in pregnancy is likely to have a greater effect than when it occurs later. In addition the immunity mechanism of a very young foetus is not very efficient compared with that of the full term baby.

If the baby is severely damaged it may die and a stillbirth or abortion follows. Slightly less damage results in the birth of a baby with congenital malformation or disease such as deafness. Sometimes the baby appears normal but deafness or other handicaps may occur either later in infancy or in childhood. The nature of damage to the baby can be as follows:

Deafness	90%
Cataract or other eye disease	50%
Congenital heart disease	40%
Psychiatric troubles	40%

Deafness is obviously the most common effect since it is present in 90 per cent of cases.

Deafness

When caused by congenital rubella this is usually due to destruction of part of the inner ear. Deafness is difficult to determine in young babies so that rubella infection probably causes more deafness than many people think. In a batch of eighty-four babies born to mothers who might have had rubella during pregnancy forty-eight babies had rubella antibodies, suggesting that they had been infected in the womb. When examined at the age of two, twenty of the infected babies had hearing problems. When they were all re-examined at the age of seven a further seven of the infected babies were found to be deaf. Thus deafness from congenital rubella may not appear until some years after birth.

In another survey three groups of children were examined:

1. Normal children of similar age groups (control group).
2. Deaf children whose mothers had had no known contact with rubella during pregnancy.

3. Deaf children whose mothers had developed rubella or been in contact with rubella during pregnancy.

The percentage of deafness in these children of different groups with the rubella antibody was as follows:

Age	*Control*	*Deaf – no known rubella contact*	*Deaf – known rubella contact*
½–2	5%	50%	95%
2–4	10%	55%	95%
4–6	25%	80%	100%

The second column shows that, as they grow older, normal children begin to acquire rubella infection and that, by the age of four to six, about 25 per cent will have been infected.

The second column shows that, although their mothers had no history of contact with rubella, more than half the babies who were deaf for no good reason were probably infected with rubella because they had rubella antibodies at the age of six months.

The last column shows that nearly all the deaf babies of mothers who had experience of rubella during pregnancy were, in fact, infected. This is shown by the fact that they had rubella antibodies at the age of six months. (By this time any antibodies from the mother that might have been present in the baby's blood will have disappeared.)

All in all it would seem that about a quarter of all babies born deaf for no good reason have suffered from rubella infection.

Heart disease

The commonest form of heart abnormality caused by congenital rubella infection is the hole between the two large chambers of the heart causing the well-known 'blue babies'. If the baby shows sign of heart failure it may be necessary to operate at birth but it is usually possible to wait until the child is several years old.

Psychiatric troubles

Two hundred and ten cases of children with congenital rubella age 8–9 were examined for psychological handicaps:

No psychiatric disorder	50%
Mentally retarded	26%
Brain malfunction	18%

Autistic	12%
Neurotic behaviour	3%

These children had been examined four years earlier when a greater number had been diagnosed as retarded—this illustrates the difficulty in assessing children with multiple handicaps. Autism occurs in about four cases per 10,000 children in all births so that prenatal rubella seems to be one, at least, of the causes of this condition as its incidence in rubella babies is several hundred times that for all births. Only about 10 per cent of congenital rubella children will be able to go to normal schools.

How often does it happen?

From the example of the children who are 'deaf without cause' it is obvious that many cases of congenital rubella are missed, especially when the mother had an attack without any illness. When a child over the age of three or four develops deafness and other defects then it is not possible at that late stage to prove that these were caused by rubella. In Britain there have been about one hundred cases reported each year for many years, despite many campaigns to reduce the incidence, but this represents only the easily diagnosable cases. In about 40 per cent of these cases the mother's infection was subclinical.

In the USA there was a widespread outbreak in 1964 and in New York City where the disease is notifiable about 1 per cent of all pregnancies were complicated with rubella and throughout the country about 30,000 children were born with handicaps because of this outbreak.

Contracting rubella infection

The virus is carried in the throat of infected persons from about a week before to a week after the rash appears (in those cases with symptoms) and the virus spreads by droplet infection to susceptible persons. The infection is rare under the age of four.

The contacts likely to transmit rubella are:

1. *Direct* e.g. living in the same house, especially brother or sister. Infection frequently follows direct contacts.
2. *Remote*, e.g. the woman is in the presence of a case for a short time such as being on the same bus. Infection does not often follow remote contacts.

3. *Indirect* e.g. visiting a house where there is a case but not meeting the case. Infection does not follow indirect contacts.
4. *Intermittent* e.g. schoolteachers. Intermittent contacts may develop infection but are difficult to deal with because there is no known date of contact; all women who come into daily contact with children should be immunized.

Screening for immunity

1. Like other infections, an attack of rubella induces the body to produce antibodies to the virus. These antibodies protect against further infections.
2. Rubella is not a very definite disease—other conditions may produce a similar rash—so that the patient's word can never be taken as to whether or not she has had rubella in the past. The presence of antibody indicates previous infection (or vaccination).
3. Thus, by detecting antibody in the woman's blood it can be confidently stated that she is immune to rubella. This is the basis of the screening test.
4. All women without antibodies should be vaccinated against rubella and retested in about six weeks time.
5. In a survey taken a few years ago of Essex school leavers the following showed immunity:

Males	73%
Females (not vaccinated)	88%
Females (vaccinated)	99%

Excretion of the virus by cases

In the ordinary disease the virus is excreted, e.g. in the saliva, for ten to fourteen days. In cases of congenital rubella the excretion is prolonged:

1. At birth 100 per cent of congenital cases excrete the virus.
2. At eight months 40 per cent excrete it.
3. At thirteen months 3 per cent still excrete it.

Thus rubella babies are highly infectious.

Vaccination against rubella

Rubella vaccine is a safe and efficient agent for producing immunity to the virus and it is given by injection. One dose is usually sufficient. It is a live vaccine and should never be given deliberately to a pregnant woman. However, this has happened many times, especially when the woman has been vaccinated just after her last period thus not yet knowing that she was pregnant. Several hundred women who were susceptible to rubella and who had been vaccinated just before or during the first three months of pregnancy elected to go ahead with their pregnancies and not a single handicapped baby was produced.

Since 1970 rubella vaccine has been offered to schoolgirls between the ages of eleven and fourteen. In 1987 this meant that the first of these schoolgirls to be vaccinated were between twenty-seven and thirty years of age. Thus most of the women of childbearing age today have been vaccinated. Many girls, however, are 'afraid of the needle' and will keep away from school when the vaccination session occurs, promising to go to their family doctor but, of course, never doing so. These girls that slip through the net, together with Asian immigrants who have never been vaccinated are mainly responsible for the one hundred or so cases of congenital rubella that still occur each year in Britain. By vaccinating both boys and girls against rubella, mumps and measles at fifteen to eighteen months rubella has been eradicated in Sweden. A similar scheme is intended by the British Department of Health.

Any woman risking or contemplating pregnancy must first ensure that she is immune to rubella!

Although a great part of my career was devoted to screening women against rubella I was never certain that this was necessary or even wise. There seems no reason why all women should not be injected with the vaccine and then screened afterwards to make sure they were immune. The reason generally given is that random vaccination would increase the number of possibly pregnant women that would be vaccinated. If we think of it, the only extra women that would be vaccinated would be those who were immune already. As we have seen, there is no evidence that even susceptible pregnant women suffer from vaccination; how much less important then would it be to vaccinate some women who were already immune. The cost of screening is not much less than the cost of vaccination and an important consideration is that, for those who feared the needle, only one injection would be needed.

Women are screened when they visit the antenatal clinic. If, before conception they were actually susceptible and have been infected in the early stages of pregnancy, nothing can be done for them when they visit the antenatal clinic. This will almost always take place after more than three months of pregnancy, by which time the rubella infection will have had its most severe effect. However, as soon as the baby has been born the mother should be vaccinated in the maternity department in order to protect her in subsequent pregnancies.

When carrying out screening tests on women from part of our district we frequently found the same women appearing on our files, susceptible in second and third pregnancies, not having been vaccinated after being found susceptible during the first pregnancy. There are obviously gross inefficiencies in the preventive medicine practices in parts of Britain.

What to do after contact with a case of rubella when pregnant

It is important that, if a pregnant woman is not certain that she is immune to rubella, she should avoid as far as she can contact with cases of rubella; she should keep away from children as far as possible but, because many patients are infected subclinically, it is not always easy to avoid contacts. If she should come into contact with a case, she should at once inform her doctor.

1. The doctor should take blood from her as soon as possible and send for testing for rubella antibody.
2. If, within a week of her exposure, antibody is present, then this antibody must have been present at the time of exposure so that she must have been immune at that time and she will not have become infected.
3. If she has no antibody, her blood must be tested three weeks later; if there is still no antibody, she is susceptible but has escaped infection.
4. If antibody appears in the second test it is probable that it is due to her having been infected as a result of the contact and she then might consider termination of the pregnancy.

A woman who comes into contact with a case of rubella during her pregnancy must at once tell her doctor.

Patients concerned must INSIST on tests being taken
A Tragedy of Errors

I recently came across a case of a woman whose daughter was born in 1978. The woman was screened for rubella at the time and found to be susceptible. She was offered rubella vaccination but refused it. She later had a second child. Some years later she went to the doctor because both she and her daughter had a rash and she had pains in the joints. The child was said to be suffering from rubella while the woman was diagnosed as suffering from 'arthritis' (pain in the joints is a common symptom of rubella in adults).

The woman's period, which was due early in April, did not arrive. Both she and her husband were aware of the danger from rubella if she was pregnant but the doctor said 'that it was virtually impossible for her to be susceptible to rubella as she had had two children previously so that she must have been screened and vaccinated if necessary on previous occasions'. As we saw earlier it is quite possible for susceptible women not to be vaccinated through several pregnancies (and this woman had refused vaccination on at least one occasion). At the end of April the woman's pregnancy test was positive and she was referred to the antenatal clinic. The letter of referral made no reference to the possibility of the woman having had rubella. It was not until in the middle of June that a specimen of blood was sent for rubella screening.

Antibody was present in the blood but it was too late to determine if it had appeared recently or was due to an infection before pregnancy. Possibly because the general practitioner had not pressed the matter, the obstetrician did not really look into the possibility of rubella infection in pregnancy or perhaps did not understand the fact that it was too late to get any useful information about the risk when, eventually, her blood was sent for examination—sixty-six days after the rash. The child was born partly blind and partly deaf.

On another occasion I had a phone call from a lady who wanted to become pregnant. Very sensibly she wanted to be screened before doing so so she rang her family doctor. The receptionist told her not to bother, just to go ahead and get pregnant and they would look after her after that!

Cytomegalovirus infection

Cytomegalovirus (CMV) infection is caused by a virus that is rarely heard of by the lay public (and even a good many doctors) but it is one that infects most people at some time during their life. In the vast majority of cases the patient will not be aware that he has been affected although in a small number of cases there is a mild illness. The virus is a member of the 'herpes group' and looks, under an electron microscope, like the one that causes chickenpox. It shares with other members of this group the ability to remain in the body long after the first illness has passed and it can sometimes reappear, so that the patient becomes infectious again.

The less hygienic the environment in which a person lives, the sooner he meets most pathogenic organisms. In Egypt, for instance, most children of two have already been infected with all three types of polio virus. Thus with CMV people coming from less hygienic environments tend to be infected earlier.

Infection in the non-pregnant

After infection the virus lives in certain white cells of the blood and 5 per cent of blood donors carry it; when their blood is transfused into patients of reduced immunity the disease may follow.

A particularly important occasion is when a baby has an exchange transfusion for Rh incompatibility; frequently a mild illness follows due to CMV infection and if the mother is susceptible she may become infected. In a similar way transfusions of blood carrying the virus and given to transplant patients whose immunity has been deliberately destroyed to prevent graft rejection may cause an illness that, fortunately, is usually mild.

Contracting cytomegalovirus infection

The lower the standards of hygiene the easier to contract infection. In Tanzania 100 per cent of children under 5 have been infected while in the UK the figure is 20 per cent. Babies under 6 months are protected by antibodies from the mother except when she has not been infected and therefore has no antibody. About 10 per cent of babies are infected in their first year, but the increase is low until about 15 when about 35 per cent will have been infected. By the age of thirty-five about 54 per cent will have been infected and will thus be immune; this compares with over 85 per cent immune to rubella.

It is believed that in Britain about 1 per cent of babies are born having been infected with CMV.

Infection of the baby

The importance of time of CMV infection is as follows:

1. *Early in pregnancy.* Infection is uncommon but it causes severe disease when it does occur, e.g. microcephaly (lack of development of

the bones of the skull, resulting in a small head and severe mental retardation).

2. *Late in pregnancy*. Infection is more common but less severe. The condition is often without symptoms – about 10 per cent of babies have them – but there may be liver infection with jaundice or a skin rash. If we follow up those babies that had symptoms we find that about 50 per cent fail to develop mentally as compared with uninfected babies and of the babies who became infected but were without symptoms 10–20 per cent will have some mental handicap.

3. *In infancy*. Because the virus is occasionally excreted by the mother who was infected in the past, a few babies are infected after birth but the effects are rarely serious.

The problem of cytomegalovirus infection

In rubella there is, in about half the cases, a rash which indicates infection of the mother. With CMV infection there is no indication of infection. As with rubella the important victims are those women who have not been infected before becoming pregnant; it is the babies of these mothers that suffer the illnesses described. Women are not screened for CMV immunity during pregnancy but they should be and termination should be offered to any who develop antibody during pregnancy, as no vaccine is available.

CMV is not a problem in the less hygienic places of the world; every woman will have been infected in childhood and will therefore be immune. In a survey in Britain it was found that 58 per cent of white women were immune compared with 90 per cent of Asian women; as a result 4 per cent of the white women became infected during pregnancy but only 2 per cent of the Asians.

It seems obvious that the average age of primary infection varies in different parts of the world; that the risk of foetal infection is higher where a larger proportion of women of childbearing age remain susceptible (i.e. have not been infected before conception); and that the problem is different for different countries. Those that work in this field maintain that there are more handicapped babies through CMV infection than through rubella.

Toxoplasmosis

This infection is caused by a tiny single celled parasite – the toxoplasma. It spends part of its life in the cat and the rest in a variety of warm blooded animals, including man. It is another of those organisms that infect a large proportion of the human population, usually without symptoms. The organisms enter certain cells of the host where they multiply, enlarging the cell which produces a thick wall around itself—a cyst. If the cyst is not disturbed it remains inactive, but if eaten by another animal (not a common occurrence in the case of human infection) it will release the small organisms within it and cause infection to the devourer. Cats are of importance in the spread of toxoplasmosis because, when they become infected, the toxoplasma undergo sexual reproduction within the cat and, for a period of 1–3 weeks before it develops immunity, the cat sheds millions of cysts in its droppings. These cysts are not directly infectious but develop into infectious forms after one to twenty-one days and need warm moist soil for this purpose.

Before the cycle within the cat was discovered, it was believed that the disease was always contracted by eating undercooked meat; however it was always difficult to explain how vegetarians contracted it.

Occurrence

The proportion of adults infected varies from country to country and is highest in the Third World, in association with cats and where food may not be well cooked. As with CMV, women who have been infected are immune and will not contract the infection during pregnancy with risk to the foetus. Thus toxoplasmosis in pregnancy is more likely to occur in hygienic countries where the number of previously infected women of childbearing age is relatively low. In Britain only about 20 per cent of women are immune, while in Paris about 80 per cent are. In Moslem countries the infection rate is low, so that, with immigrant Moslem workers in Paris, the risk of toxoplasmosis in pregnancy is much greater than for native *Parisiennes*. When a woman is infected during pregnancy the infection is passed to the baby in about 50 per cent of cases.

The infection

If infection of the mother occurs early in pregnancy the child is less likely to become affected, but if it does it is often severely damaged, with irreparable brain damage, eye damage and a high risk of mental defect. Infection of the baby late in pregnancy is more likely to happen but the infection is nearly always mild with no permanent damage occurring.

Avoiding toxoplasmosis

The logical suggestion is to bring women up in the presence of cats so that infection occurs early in life, well before pregnancy; however, during pregnancy they should keep away from cats, especially young ones. If they cannot avoid caring for cats, they should at least wear gloves when cleaning out cat litter. They should also wear gloves when gardening because there is the possibility that the soil may be contaminated by cat droppings.

Patients may be screened for immunity and in a perfect world all women would be screened before pregnancy. Those with no antibody should be screened monthly for the first four months of pregnancy and any found to have become infected during this period should be offered termination.

The incidence of congenital toxoplasmosis varies from country to country:

	Per 1,000 live births
Germany	5
France	3
Britain	0.25
USA	1.6

Obviously the risk in Britain is slight.

Future work on infections during pregnancy

Before we do anything we ought to know the size of the problems facing us:

1. What proportion of pregnant women are susceptible.
2. What proportion become infected in pregnancy.
3. How often congenital infection occurs in Britain.

The best way of tackling these issues would be to encourage the monitoring of women throughout pregnancy; they should be screened for immunity to rubella, CMV and toxoplasmosis. If there could be a tie-up with family planning clinics and pregnancy testing units, screening could be started before pregnancy. In this way we would be able to get a real picture of the relative importances of infection during pregnancy and not just speculations as at present. Unfortunately it would cost money!

As far as rubella is concerned, we know the risks. Effort should be concentrated on vaccination, not screening. Every schoolgirl should be vaccinated twice, at a year's interval. Women wanting to become pregnant should be vaccinated and then, preferably, tested for the success of the vaccination before becoming pregnant. Alternatively, the Department of Health's new proposal to vaccinate all children of both sexes early in life—as is done in the USA where there has been a substantial decrease in the incidence of congenital rubella as a result—is sure to improve the situation.

Listeriosis

It is not clear why the group of organisms that include *L. monocytogenes* was named after Lord Lister, the surgeon who made surgery safer for patients by introducing antiseptic methods. The second part of its name arises from its ability to increase the number of certain white cells—monocytes—in the blood of infected rabbits, rodents and man but not in other animals it infects.

The organism is very common in the environment, in soil, mouldy fodder, etc., and from these sources it is able to contaminate various foodstuffs, especially salads. The organism resembles *Cl. welchii* in its widespread distribution and the fact that it can only infect man under certain circumstances. It has the ability to multiply at refrigerator temperatures but is killed easily by heat.

The organism was not recognized until 1933 and reports of human infections were very rare at first. It soon became clear that pregnant women were at greatest risk, possibly because of their reduced immunity. The organism appears to remain with the patient, so that two or more successive miscarriages may occur. It has been suggested that Queen Anne (1702–14) became chronically infected; she had seventeen pregnancies which included eleven abortions, one stillbirth, two neonatal deaths and a child dying from what seem to be the result of congenital infection of the brain.

In humans the commonest result of infection is miscarriage and, if the child survives the pregnancy, it may develop fatal meningitis after three weeks or so. Older people may also develop fatal meningitis.

Avoiding listeriosis

It is very difficult to give any useful advice on avoiding an organism so abundant in the environment and which so rarely causes infection. The infection is still rare but, possibly because the organism is looked for more often than formerly, the number of diagnosed cases is increasing. In 1988 there were 115 cases associated with pregnancy and about 1 in 4 resulted in foetal or neonatal deaths.

It would seem wise for pregnant women to avid ripe, soft cheeses, which quite frequently contain many listeria organisms. Monitoring of cook-chilled foods and ready-to-eat poultry might be useful, while ready-cooked foods should be reheated so as to maintain a core temperature of 70°C for at least 2 minutes and the food should be served immediately.

Chickenpox

As we have already seen, when chickenpox occurs in a mother less than five days before delivery the baby will have no maternal antibody and may be infected, either in the womb or shortly after delivery. Thus such a baby should always be given ready-made antibody soon after delivery. As about 8 per cent of pregnant women lack chickenpox antibody and are thus susceptible, we would expect quite a few infections in pregnancy.

It has been already mentioned that the chickenpox virus causes chickenpox in children but remains in the body and in later life may cause shingles. On a few occasions when a pregnant woman has developed chickenpox early in pregnancy the baby has become infected but sustains little damage except that it develops shingles in childhood rather than in old age.

AIDS

We shall be talking more about this infection later but it must be mentioned here in relation to pregnancy. If a woman who has been infected with the HIV virus becomes pregnant there are two risks:

1. She may pass the infection on to the baby (50 per cent).
2. Her pregnancy makes it more likely that she will develop the disease.

A number of cases of AIDS in children of infected mothers (mainly intravenous drug addicts) have occurred in Britain, but it is not clear how many infections have been truly congenital and how many caused by contact, e.g. breast feeding after birth (1987). Sometimes the mother has been the partner of a man who has acquired the infection through homosexual contact; sometimes she might be a drug addict and sometimes married to a haemophiliac who has contracted the infection from the clotting factor used for the treatment of his haemophilia. A woman who is aware that she has been infected by the HIV virus should think very carefully before becoming pregnant; if she does decide to, then she has to consider the risk of passing on the HIV in breast milk. It is not clear at present whether the advantages of breast feeding outweigh the added risk of HIV infection.

Hepatitis B

This is another infection we shall be discussing later. If a baby is born to a woman suffering from this acute disease – i.e. the woman is actually ill and not merely carrying the virus – the baby should be given ready-made antibody and also vaccinated at birth to reduce its chances of becoming infected.

Chlamydia

These are rather like small bacteria and cause a variety of infectious diseases including 'parrot disease' (psittacosis). Type A chlamydia usually infect the eyes and the genitalia. In the male they occasionally cause a discharge but often there are no symptoms. Infection is through sexual intercourse and in women it is usually the cervix – the neck of the womb – that harbours the infection. This infection may be symptom-free or may cause moderate damage to the cervix together with a vaginal discharge. When a woman with such a cervical infection is delivered, the baby is squeezed through the cervix and this intimate contact results in infection of the baby's eyes. As a result the baby's eyes begin to discharge five to twelve days after birth. The condition will usually clear up without treatment after a few weeks but, if treated with tetracycline, it will disappear after a few days.

Gonococcal infection

We shall be talking about gonorrhoea as a sexually transmitted disease later but it is worth remembering that, before the advent of antibiotics, the infection of the baby's eyes with the gonococcus at birth was the commonest cause of blindness in children. The mode of infection is very like that of chlamydia but with gonorrhoea the man usually has a profuse discharge. The organism lodges in the mother's cervix and the baby is infected while being born. Before the days of antibiotics every district midwife carried in her bag a bottle of dilute silver nitrate solution for putting drops into the baby's eyes at birth as a routine—Crede's method of preventing gonococcal ophthalmia. Today the condition is almost unknown in Britain.

Infection by the herpes virus

We shall be talking later about genital herpes infection. It is sufficient to say here that when active vaginal infection by the herpes virus is present at the time of labour there is a real risk of the baby becoming infected. To avoid this it is wise to deliver the baby the other way—by carrying out a Caesarian section.

There are many other infections that can complicate pregnancy or childbirth but few are harmful to the foetus. For instance, a survey to assess the effect of influenza infection during pregnancy showed only a significant excess of male babies in the women who had been infected—it is not suggested that this be used as a method of controlling the sex of offspring!

Artificial insemination by donor

Human artificial insemination by donor (AID) is becoming more popular, not only in cases of sterility but also where unmarried women wish to become pregnant without the intrusion of a man. Recently some cases of foetal infection have occurred when the donor was not properly screened. Cases of infection caused by cytomegalovirus and by herpes simplex have been recorded; these are particularly unpleasant infections for the foetus. More recently a donor who had HIV antibody without knowing about it at the time infected 2 of 4 recipients. Thus the possibility of AIDS complicating AID must always be considered.

FIVE

Chiefly Concerning Children

Measles

Measles is still regarded by many people as an inevitable disease – a part of childhood – but it can leave serious consequences and occasionally kill. *It is a disease that can and ought to be prevented by routine vaccination of all children.*

It was earlier called 'mezils' and thought to be a mild form of smallpox and was only distinguished as a disease in its own right about 1620. In the seventeenth century deaths from measles in London varied from two to 150 per year. Between 1838 and 1842 the mean annual death rates for various common diseases were:

	Per million	*Today's projected figures*
Diphtheria and scarlet fever	797	40,000
Measles	539	25,000
Whooping cough	504	25,000

The last column indicates the number who would have died if the population of Britain had been the size it is today.

After 1850 the death rate for measles began to fall but as recently as 1955 there were 176 deaths. Part of the reason for the fall was the introduction of antibiotics but, as with some other epidemic diseases, improved hygiene and nutrition and the trend towards smaller families plus the fact that measles is more dangerous for small babies all seem to be important factors.

The disease

An attack of measles starts with the patient feeling unwell for two to four days. A high temperature, vomiting and sometimes diarrhoea may occur; there is always a dry cough. The rash first appears behind the ears after three to five days of illness and over the next two or three days spreads down the body. The spots are large and dark red, fairly flat and tending to join together to form a blotchy rash. It fades from the top and leaves some skin staining for about a week. Once the rash appears the temperature begins to return to normal and the patient starts to feel better. About 8 per cent of patients develop complications; chest and ear infections, caused by bacteria, are the commonest.

Measles is one of those diseases where there are no carriers and no subclinical disease so that infection is always from another case of measles; however, infection may be contracted from early cases where the rash has not yet appeared. The virus is inhaled and settles on the lining of the air passages. Here it enters the cells and begins to multiply. After about ten to fourteen days (the incubation period) there is sufficient virus to invade the blood stream; in this way it is carried all over the body and can affect any part. The rash is the effect of the virus on the skin cells. It can also affect the lungs, intestine, ear and brain.

In some countries the disease is very severe and there are occasions when it has been introduced into populations that have never before been in contact with it where a large number of people in the community have died following infection. In rural Africa the disease is very severe and 6–26 per cent of those contracting it die. When introduced into Fiji in 1875 25 per cent of the population died.

Measles infection illustrates well the fact that, once the body's cells have been affected by a virus, many bacteria, not normally dangerous, can enter the damaged tissue and cause secondary infection. Thus, although antibiotics do not affect viruses, they are sometimes used in virus infections to treat or prevent secondary infections by bacteria.

Prevention

A live vaccine is used – that is, a strain of measles virus which has been grown under circumstances that make it unable to cause illness. It should be given before the second year of life and it is very effective. In the USA measles immunization is obligatory before entry into many schools and in some states this has led to the virtual elimination of the disease. In Britain the uptake is only about 50 per cent which is not sufficient to effectively reduce the incidence.

Mumps

There are a large number of different viruses included in the group called myxoviruses. One of these is influenza and another is mumps. The word 'mump' is an old word meaning to mope but it is no more applicable to this disease than to many others. Mumps is a disease that can occur without symptoms, especially in infants, and it may be from these unsuspected cases that most clinical infections arise. Over 95 per cent of people will have had the infection before they die. The incubation period – that is, the interval between infection occurring and the patient becoming ill – is two to three weeks. We recognize typical mumps by the swelling of the parotid salivary glands in the angles behind the jaw and below the ear; the appearance is characteristic.

As with the measles virus, mumps virus is inhaled and multiplies in the lining of the upper air passages. When it has multiplied sufficiently it invades the bloodstream and is carried all over the body. It tends to affect the salivary glands most often, where it damages one side only in about 25 per cent of cases, but it can also affect the testes and the ovaries. Although some damage is caused to the testes, sterility rarely follows, contrary to popular belief. The coverings of the brain may also be invaded, when meningitis follows. Quite often meningitis is the only indication of mumps infection; it is not usually serious but may rarely cause permanent deafness.

A live vaccine is available for prevention of the disease; it is very effective and used extensively in the USA and Scandinavian countries but, in view of the generally mild course of the disease, it is not used widely in Britain. However, the former Department of Health and Social Security in Britain recently introduced vaccination of infants of fifteen to eighteen months with a combined rubella, measles and mumps vaccine.

Chickenpox (varicella)

The word 'pox', used frequently to describe skin rashes, simply refers to the 'pocks' or holes left behind as scars. The two classic 'poxes' are the smallpox (variola) and the Great Pox or syphilis because both of these diseases are noted for the scars and deformities of the skin that they leave behind. Chickenpox rarely leaves serious scars so that it is probably because of the resemblance of the rash to that of smallpox that gives it the 'pox' part of its name. The 'chicken' part comes not from the bird but probably from the resemblance of the little blisters to chick peas. A number of similar virus infections affect animals, so that we may encounter canary pox, mouse pox and even buffalo pox!

Except in the newborn and in children with diminished immunity chickenpox is an extremely mild disease. Hence there is doubt if there is any virtue in isolating patients, except for the fact that these days there are more children with impaired immunity in the community and these children might be severely affected if they contracted the infection. Usually chickenpox is only about as severe as the common cold and at least 75 per cent of people suffer from it at some time or other.

The virus that causes the infection is very like those causing herpes and cytomegalovirus infections and glandular fever; under the electron microscope these viruses are indistinguishable.

They have other things in common too. After the illness the virus remains in the body, presumably for life. The viruses of herpes and chickenpox live in certain nerve cells, while those of cytomegalovirus disease and glandular fever live in certain white cells of the blood and some other cells. The result of this persistent infection is that, under conditions of stress, the viruses can emerge from their hiding places and cause further illness.

The virus of chickenpox lives in the bodies of certain sensory nerves – those that look after 'skin feeling' – either of the trunk or of the head and neck. When the patient comes under stress, such as irradiation – or sometimes for no known reason – the virus migrates down the nerve fibres to the skin where it sets up a localized attack of chickenpox; this is the well-known condition of 'shingles'. Because each nerve supplies the feeling to a small but well-defined territory, the distribution of the rash of shingles also covers a definite area, usually a band round the chest or abdomen. It is usually on one side only but when on both there is no truth in the belief that when the two bands meet in the middle the patient dies!

However, shingles is a very painful disease and its effects may persist for months or years in the form of a neuralgic pain and extreme tenderness, especially to the pressure of clothes. When the sensory nerve to the eye is affected severe secondary infection may occur with the possibility of blindness. When the nerve supplying the ear is affected there is severe pain in the external ear, sometimes deafness and sometimes paralysis of that side of the face.

The rash of chickenpox appears after an incubation period of about three weeks. It begins on the body and spreads to the face and limbs. The spots are flat to begin with but soon become little blisters. These soon burst and crust. Each day for about a week new crops appear so that, at the same time, one can see flat and raised spots, blisters and crusts. The skin usually heals without trouble. When adults catch chickenpox their condition is usually more serious than that of infected children and they run the risk of developing pneumonia. I have seen two fatal cases: one in an expectant mother and one in a recently delivered woman, coincidentally at the same time and almost in the same place.

Chickenpox can be severe in a newborn baby. Therefore, when a mother develops the infection just before labour it is important to give the baby specific antiserum as soon as possible, as the mother must have lacked antibody to have contracted the infection. There is usually no need to treat with antibiotics, etc. unless the patient's immunity is deficient, in which case antiviral drugs are needed.

Scarlet fever

Scarlet fever is a throat infection caused by a bacterium called a streptococcus. 'Streptos' is Greek for a spiral and 'coccus' means a small round bacterium. These bacteria grow in chains and under the microscope they look vaguely like spirals. Most of the streptococci are quite harmless but a few can cause a number of human and animal diseases. As well as causing throat infection they can infect the skin (erysipelas) and were also responsible for many deaths due to infection following childbirth (puerperal sepsis), as in the Semmelweiss affair described in Chapter 3. Before the days of penicillin, streptococcal infections were very frightening, with death from 'blood poisoning' often following a minor injury. Even today the same condition, more formally known as bacteraemia, occurs too frequently. In a British hospital in the 1980s, there were forty cases in seven years caused by the streptococcus and 35 per cent of the patients died.

Scarlet fever is an old disease in Britain. (The phrase was also used to signify a liking for soldiers on the part of certain ladies; the soldiers wore red coats in those days.) The severity of scarlet fever has altered over the years; in 1863 the death rate per million children under fifteen was 4,000. Then, from 1866 the mortality declined and in 1953 there were only twenty-seven deaths. Today a death from scarlet fever must be rare indeed.

In the older accounts it is sometimes difficult to decide whether the writer is talking about diphtheria or scarlet fever as they were often confused. However, when the two were separated, it became obvious that scarlet fever was much less dangerous than diphtheria. During the first third of this century two complications of scarlet fever were more serious than the infection itself. These were rheumatic fever and acute nephritis.

Rheumatic fever

Of all the obscure saints, St Vitus must be one of the most obscure. It is known that he was born in Sicily and martyred by the Romans but how and why he became converted to Christianity, how he offended the Romans to the point of martyrdom, and why after his death he became the patron saint of those who have difficulty in controlling their movements is far from clear. He is, indeed, the patron saint of epileptics and those suffering from chorea – the sinuous, snaky movements of those suffering from rheumatic fever. The fact that he is the patron saint of dancers as well is also of interest and, by a 'folkloric' reversal of logic, I remember as a child often being told 'to stop fidgeting or you'll get St Vitus's Dance!'

St Vitus's Dance comes not from a propensity for fidgeting but is one of the symptoms of rheumatic fever, which has hardly anything to do with 'rheumatism' but is a complication of streptococcal infection. The other symptoms are a fever, pains in the joints and damage to the heart. The first three troubles pass but the damage to the heart progresses. As well as damaging the heart muscle, the disease causes inflammation of the surfaces of the valves that prevent the back flow of blood into the heart. The commonest to be affected is the mitral valve, which prevents the backflow of blood from the aorta. This valve has two cusps that separate to allow the blood to flow out of the heart and then come together to prevent backflow. If their surfaces become inflamed there is a tendency for them to stick together at their edges, thus reducing the size of the hole the blood has to pass through to reach the body; this causes a damming back of the blood in the lungs and a shortage to the rest of the body. The condition is known as 'mitral stenosis'.

When I first qualified mitral stenosis was a common cause of fatal heart disease in young people (a girlfriend of mine suffered from it in the early 1940s – she must have died long ago). Today it occurs rarely in Britain, mainly because the prompt use of antibiotics in streptococcal infections prevents the emergence of rheumatic fever. Also the use of prophylactic penicillin on the few who do develop the complication seems to prevent deterioration of the heart. Finally, if the mitral valve becomes affected, it is nowadays a matter of routine to repair it or insert an artificial valve.

In the Third World, however, rheumatic fever is still as important a disease as it was in Britain forty or fifty years ago.

Acute nephritis

Acute nephritis is another complication of streptococcal infection and affects the kidney. It occurs some time after the streptococcal infection and consists of damage to the small filtering tubes of the kidney as a result of a hypersensitivity reaction. This leads to failure to excrete water from the body. As a result the body becomes 'waterlogged', with puffiness around the eyes and ankles. The condition clears up in a week or so but can lead to permanent damage of the kidneys, leading to early death. This condition is now rare in Britain but still occurs in the Third World.

Diphtheria

While the severity of scarlet fever has waxed and waned, that of diphtheria has remained constant, with a high death rate. It was not common in Britain until about 1855 but by 1859 it had become very common. It was known as the 'Boulougne sore throat'; in 1855–6 there were epidemics in several parts of Britain including Billericay in Essex and in 1859 there were nearly 10,000 deaths in England and Wales.

Diphtheria is an infection in which a toxin is formed. That is to say the bacteria multiply in the throat, causing inflammation and the formation of a membrane, but do not invade the rest of the body. As the bacteria multiply they produce a powerful toxin or poison that travels throughout the body via the bloodstream and is able to paralyse certain muscles.

One of the characteristic appearances of diphtheria in the early days was a child with a sore throat and 'footdrop' – the inability to bend the foot upwards. Later the small muscles of the eye would be affected so that the patient could not focus his eyes. If the heart became paralysed the patient died.

In the early days of immunology it was soon found that, by injecting horses with some of the liquid in which the diphtheria bacilli had grown, the horses produced antitoxin – a substance that neutralized the toxin – so that it no longer caused death.

Antitoxin made from horses was used to treat cases of diphtheria from 1895 onwards. However, since the antitoxin contained horse protein, one or two deaths from hypersensitivity occurred before it was realized that it was necessary to first give a tiny dose to test the patient's sensitivity to the protein before giving the whole dose.

Antitoxin was also used to protect children who had been in contact with cases of diphtheria; in New York in 1895–1900 more than 6,000 contacts were given antitoxin and less than 1 per cent caught the disease. In 1913 attempts were made to actively immunize children with a mixture of toxin and antitoxin and over 70 per cent were rendered immune; but in Vienna in 1924 seven children died after injection of the toxin/antitoxin mixture because for various reasons the toxin was not completely neutralized.

In 1922, in Britain, some culture medium containing diphtheria toxin was stored in vats that had contained formaldehyde (formalin) and it was found that this altered the toxin so that it did not cause illness but did produce immunity. The altered toxin was called 'toxoid', which was used widely from 1925 onward in the USA for immunizing children. (See Figure 5.1.) It was not for another fifteen years and after the deaths of thousands of children that the British Ministry of Health launched a vaccination campaign in the early 1940s and that against stiff opposition from the Antivivisection Society.

Figure 5.1 Toxin and toxoid

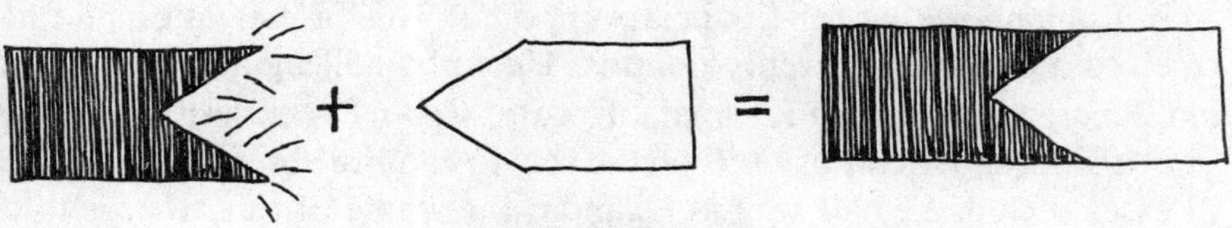

By the late 1930s there were no longer any cases of diphtheria in any of the major Canadian cities but in 1943, when I was a resident in a fever hospital in northern England, I quite often admitted as many as twelve cases of diphtheria in one day. In 1947 I went into the army and the last case of diphtheria I saw before joining up was my own sister. When I came back from Africa in 1949 diphtheria was a rare disease and I have not personally seen a case since.

Diphtheria can be prevented by vaccination which is given as part of the 'triple vaccine'; this also contains tetanus and whooping cough vaccine and is begun in the third month of life. A high acceptance rate is needed if the disease is to remain as rare as it is today and this is illustrated by an outbreak that occurred in a large mental hospital near Colchester in Essex some years ago. The necessity for keeping up the vaccination status of the patients had been forgotten for years and, when a diphtheria carrier was inadvertently admitted, there were about twenty cases of diphtheria among the patients and staff, with several deaths.

Glandular fever

Glandular fever is a very common disease but it is not always recognized. The story of the discovery of its cause goes back to the end of the Second World War. A young Irishman, Denis Burkitt, attempted to join the army as a surgeon but, as he had lost the sight of one eye in an accident, he was not accepted. Later he was allowed to join up and was sent to the hospital at Kampala in Uganda where he was one of the senior surgeons.

After the war he remained at Kampala and among the patients brought to him were children with horrific growths of the face, mainly in the lower jaw. He became interested in these cases, having never seen anything like them before, and he wondered about their cause and distribution.

He became so interested that he wrote to the Medical Research Council in England asking for financial support for his investigation and he received a cheque for twenty pounds. He and a colleague drove, in an old American car, from Kampala down to Cape Town, visiting all the small towns and their hospitals on the way to enquire about the existence of cases such as he had seen in Uganda; the whole of this story is told in a fascinating book, *The Great Safari*. After receiving a few more pounds from the MRC Burkitt then organized a postal survey, writing to all the hospitals in Africa about these cases.

As far as treatment was concerned, Burkitt found that surgery was useless because so much of the growth was mixed up with the normal tissue. He felt that the best form of treatment would be with x-rays, but there was a snag here because there was not at that time a suitable machine available between Cairo and Capetown. As most missionaries need to be, Burkitt was an accomplished scrounger and he persuaded drug representatives to get their firms to send him all their samples of anti-cancer drugs. He was not very optimistic of the result as these drugs usually needed to be taken over long periods to be effective with the cancers he had come across so far. However, to his delight he found that a single dose was usually enough to persuade the growths to shrink. This was ideal because most of his patients were brought to him from the bush, which was where they tended to disappear back to after a single dose.

The next part of the story came when Burkitt came home on leave and gave a lecture at the Middlesex Hospital in London. He spoke at length about these growths, which were now called Burkitt's lymphoma. In the audience there was a young research worker called Michael Epstein, who was interested in cancers that were caused by micro-organisms. These were known in animals but, so far, no definite infectious cancer for man had been discovered.

In giving the results of his research, Burkitt said that the lymphoma appeared only in areas that were warm and damp and that no cases were found near the Sahara, for instance. Epstein at once felt this might be because a microbe was the cause and he asked Burkitt to send him some tissue from some cases. Much later this was possible and after a number of tests it was decided to grow the cells from this tumour in a bottle – the method, called tissue culture, has revolutionized the culture of viruses over the last forty years. These cells were eventually persuaded to grow and, as the two people working with them were Michael Epstein and Yvonne Barr, the bottle was labelled 'EB'. These cells became known as Epstein–Barr cells.

Having grown the cells and carried out various other tests, Epstein decided to cut very thin sections and look at them under an electron microscope. To his amazement he saw, among the cells, small viruses identical in appearance with those that caused herpes infection and chickenpox.

The presence of these viruses at once suggested that they were the cause of the tumours in the African children so that it became important to find out what viruses they were. There is a way of identifying unknown viruses by treating them with antibody produced by injecting animals with known viruses and attaching a fluorescent dye to this antibody. Thus if an unknown virus treated with antibody produced by injecting chickenpox virus into an animal glowed green under the microscope then the unknown virus was that of chickenpox and it would not glow in this way if treated with antibody made using the herpes virus. This test was applied to the EB cells using antibodies to all the known members of the herpes family of viruses, both human and animal types. Not one of them gave a positive reaction and at this point the investigation seemed to have run out of steam.

At this stage the American marines came galloping in, figuratively speaking, in the person of Professor W. Henle and his wife, Gertrude. They were interested in viruses and in the methods used by Epstein. They tested the cells against all sorts of antibodies to viruses without result. Then they used plain serum from ordinary people instead of antibody raised in animals. They were very surprised to find that *over 50 per cent of normal people* had in their blood antibodies to this unknown virus.

This was very confusing since a virus isolated from the cells of a cancer that occurred almost exclusively in central Africa – a virus that was believed to cause this condition – had made contact with over half the population of the USA at some time or other!

The situation remained like this for some time until one day Elaine Hutner, one of the technicians in the Henle's laboratory, became ill, with a sore throat and swollen glands. Her blood was examined, certain tests were carried out and there was no doubt that she was suffering from glandular fever. Now Elaine's serum had been tested, together with that from all the other workers in that laboratory, and it was one of the specimens that failed to produce fluorescence in the EB cells.

When Elaine returned to work her serum was tested again and it was found that the test was now positive – the cells fluoresced with her serum. Thus it seemed probable that the virus present in the EB was the one that caused glandular fever. This has been established without doubt by many other tests taken before and after glandular fever. We now know that glandular fever is a world-wide disease but we are little nearer to finding out why it takes the form of these growths on some children in central Africa.

The illness

Glandular fever is an illness in which the patient suffers from enlarged lymph glands all over the body, sore throat, temperature, headache and various other general symptoms of infection including loss of appetite and nausea. A film of the blood shows a large increase of certain white cells and there are other blood tests for the disease. The disease is caused by the EB virus which infects certain of the white cells of the blood and, when these die, further virus is released which infects further cells. Because the surfaces of these white cells have been altered by the infection they are regarded as foreign by other white cells. The latter now multiply so that they can destroy the 'foreign' cells. The great increase in these white cells accounts for their increase in the blood film and also for the enlarged lymph glands.

Many babies and young children become infected early in life and in these cases there is little sign of illness; it is in the older child and young adult that the full picture of glandular fever appears. The virus remains continuously present in the body for the rest of the patient's life and, in theory, he remains infectious all his life. The virus is present in the throat for up to eighteen months after recovery and intermittently present in all who have recovered, about 10 per cent being positive at any one time.

Although glandular-fever causes little illness in the younger age groups, it is a very common cause of illness in those such as students in the fifteen to twenty-five age range who are grouped together. It does not cause epidemics and there is no point in isolating patients. There is no need for any special treatment as the patient usually recovers in two to three weeks. He needs be kept in bed only when he feels like it but, as the spleen may be enlarged, violent exercise or the lifting of heavy weights should be avoided for a few weeks. In a very few cases weakness and depression persists for a long period and there is still debate about whether or not this infection may give rise to permanent weakness and lassitude.

Whooping cough

Whooping was originally spelt 'hooping' and is still pronounced that way by everyone except for an old friend of mine of Russian extraction who actually pronounces the 'w'. Another term once used was 'chincough', which had nothing to do with the chin but came from old German 'to gasp'.

The disease

Whooping cough affects children from a few months upwards. It may also effect older people; on one occasion a grandfather brought a child up for a swab to be taken and, on hearing the older person cough, a swab was taken from him and found to contain the causative bacterium, *Bordetella pertussis. Pertussis* is the Latinized name for the infection but it just means cough.

The incubation period is seven to ten days and the infection begins as a catarrhal illness with lots of snuffling, sometimes with the symptoms of croup. After ten days or so the characteristic spasmodic cough appears. The linings of the air passages become swollen and obstructed with mucus so that the child cannot breathe out. He coughs to remove the obstruction again and again until his lungs are empty of air and then needs to take a long deep breath which accounts for the whoop. Thus the whoop is made on inspiration.

The disease is more often fatal in children under a year old and may leave permanent lung damage or affect the brain. It is a severe and wearing disease, both for the baby and the mother and it is sometimes worthwhile to admit the child to hospital in order to give the mother a rest.

Incidence

In Britain, there were more than 4,000 deaths from whooping cough in 1928 and 678 deaths in 1948; since 1961 there have been about thirty deaths each year. However, it is difficult to determine the actual number of cases. In 1977 there were about 17,000 cases notified in Britain, although only a few were confirmed bacteriologically. Perhaps the true number is ten times the number notified. It is estimated that there are about 750,000 deaths from whooping cough every year in Asia, Africa and South America.

Avoiding whooping cough

There are various ways to avoid whooping cough:

1. Vaccination. There has been more controversy about whooping cough vaccine than any other. No vaccines are completely safe; I have seen several deaths following needless typhoid vaccinations. The most harmful condition that whooping cough vaccine is said to produce is brain damage. This can occur in young babies through many causes and, if a large proportion receive whooping cough vaccine, there must be a few that will contract brain damage soon after the vaccination for reasons unrelated to vaccination.

There is a team of doctors in London that investigate all cases of brain damage in Britain. On one occasion they went to examine such a case in the Midlands and on the mantelpiece was an appointment card for the child to have his whooping cough vaccination the following week. If his illness had happened two weeks later the vaccine would have been blamed.

There is a system of payments to parents who are able to make out a convincing case that their child's brain damage was due to vaccination and this is likely to persuade the parents of any brain-damaged baby that, even if the possibility is remote, the damage was indeed caused by vaccination. When such a selective system exists it is bound to lead to bias in diagnosis, especially on the part of parents, and a payment for all cases of brain damage, whatever the cause, would seem a fairer system. A large survey has been going on for several years in one of the health regions near London and so far no serious reactions to whooping cough vaccination have been detected.

In order to protect themselves from criticism should something go wrong, doctors and nurses have in the past been rather too liberal in rejecting children for vaccination. As a result, many children, who may have been rejected because of a mild allergy, have developed the disease and suffered severe complications, since these were the children most likely to suffer worst from the infection.

Any child who appears healthy at the time and has no family history of fits, epilepsy or convulsions should be vaccinated.

2. Vaccination should be carried out early in life; it has been suggested that one injection of vaccine should be given at the end of each of the first three months of life.

3. Booster doses of vaccine may be given to older children when a new baby is expected in the household.

4. When an older child in a family with a young baby develops the disease, both the child and the baby may be given an antibiotic such as erythromycin to both treat the one and protect the other.

SIX

Infections of the Brain and Nerves

There are three main components in the nervous system: the brain, the spinal cord and the nerves.

The brain

The brain is the great biological computer and is housed in the skull which protects it from damage. (See Figure 6.1.) The base of the skull is pierced with a variety of holes for the passage of nerves and blood vessels to other parts of the body. To provide further protection the brain is contained in a bag of fluid which buffers it against blows. The linings of this bag are known as the meninges; when infection occurs

Figure 6.1 The brain within the skull

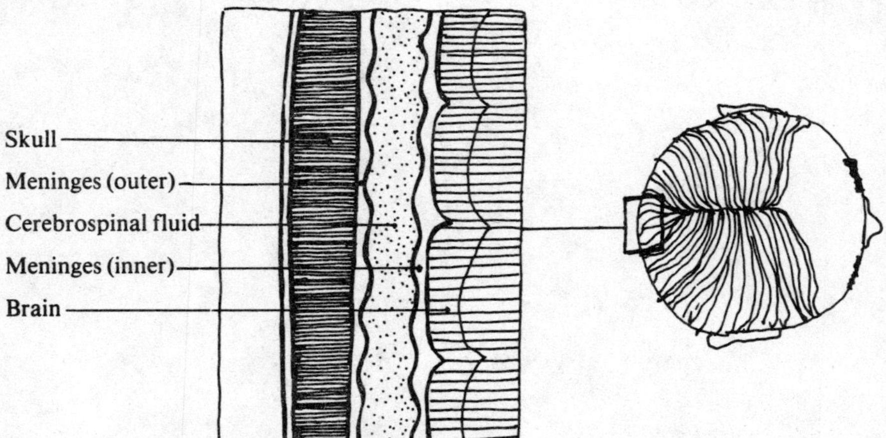

in this area it does not usually begin in the brain itself but on the meninges, causing meningitis. Infection of the meninges has severe secondary effects on the brain because the pressure generated distorts and blocks the passages through which the cerebrospinal fluid flows and may constrict blood vessels so that the areas of the brain supplied by these vessels may die; however, if the infection is treated early permanent brain damage can be avoided. The fluid that protects the brain (the cerebrospinal fluid – CSF) flows down round the outside of the spinal cord and can be sampled by inserting a needle through the skin and between the vertebrae in the lumbar region (about the middle of the back) and through the outer membrane. Examination of that sample of fluid allows us to determine the condition of the fluid over the brain. If there are pus cells in the CSF then meningitis is present.

The spinal cord

The spinal cord is a bundle of nerve fibres with their necessary cells that passes down the back; the nerve fibres are protected by the vertebrae, which provide a flexible but solid cover so that the cord does not become kinked or damaged in any other way. If the patient sits up and bends forward, it is just possible to insert a needle between two vertebrae at a point where the spinal cord has ended but where the canal containing the cerebrospinal fluid is still present. In this way the CSF may be safely sampled.

The cells of the nerves lie close by the vertebral column and may supply a permanent home to herpes simplex and chickenpox viruses. Some cells are damaged by the poliomyelitis virus and this is the cause of the paralysis.

The nerves

To remind us that we are still segmented animals like earthworms we possess a series of very similar components, for instance the ribs, the vertebrae and the nerves. The latter are given off at intervals from the spinal cord and pass out usually through gaps between the vertebrae. Many of the nerves are quite large and divide as they run outwards to the arms or downward to the legs. There are two main types:

1. The motor nerves carry messages from the brain or cord *to* the muscles instructing them to contract or relax.
2. The sensory nerves carry messages *from* the skin and other areas to the brain or cord, indicating pain, heat, touch and also position in space.

Damage to a *motor* nerve or its cell will cause paralysis while damage to a *sensory* nerve will cause loss of feeling or of balance.

Meningitis

One of the best-known infections of the nervous system is meningitis – the infection of the membranes covering the brain. In the past this has been a frightening diseases with a high mortality rate and a tendency to leave survivors with severe mental problems. Today the use of antibiotics has reduced the mortality and vaccines are likely to be available in the not too distant future to prevent the condition. As with many diseases, the impact on the Third World is much greater than in the West; there are nearly always large epidemics occurring in Africa just south of the Sahara and a recent letter to the *Lancet* talks of a large epidemic in Saudi Arabia involving 700 cases.

Organisms responsible for meningitis

Many different types of organism can cause meningitis:

1. Bacteria
   Meningococci – meningococcal meningitis
   H. influenzae – influenzal meningitis
   Str. pneumoniae – pneumococcal meningitis

These are the commonest causes in Britain, where there are about 400 cases of each per year; however, recently the incidence of meningococcal meningitis has doubled.

2. Viruses
   Coxsackie
   ECHO
   Mumps
   Herpes

Meningitis caused by viruses is rarely serious apart from rare cases of herpes virus meningitis. The coxsackie and ECHO viruses tend to cause a variety of symptoms; not only do the symptoms include meningitis, but also gastric upsets, pains in the muscles and sometimes a rash occur in mild epidemics, one type one year and another the next (there are thirty-four types of ECHO viruses, twenty-four types of Coxsackie A and six of Coxsackie B at the last count!).

3. Amoebae

Naegleri fowleri

These infections are very rare but often fatal. This organism caused a fatal case of meningitis in Bath some years ago and was found in the spa waters. This source of infection was eradicated by the large amount of rebuilding and excavation that has taken place there over recent years; the spa waters are now pure!

The illness

A classic picture is a child who is unable to kiss his knees because his neck is stiff and painful, who is vomiting, who has a severe headache and who cannot stand a bright light. Some cases of meningococcal meningitis have a rash—once again we have an organism that multiples in the throat and then invades the blood, affecting first the skin ('Spotted fever') and then the meninges. Sometimes the rash appears several days before the meningitis and sometimes there is no meningitis, just the rash and severe illness.

Diagnosis of meningitis

A lumbar puncture is performed and the CSF examined microscopically for pus cells and bacteria. It is also cultured and any organism grown is tested for susceptibility towards different antibiotics.

Prevention of meningitis

Meningococcal meningitis behaves rather oddly. The organism is not uncommon and can be found in the throats of up to 10 per cent of normal people; but sometimes a husband and wife will contract the disease within a few days of each other and at other times cases will cluster in a certain district for no known reason. Because of the limited degree of apparent infectivity it is recommended that close contacts of cases be given antibiotics as soon as the condition is diagnosed.

When young people are grouped together infectious diseases tend to be picked up by the susceptible, as in the 'back-to-school' situation; on a larger scale, for example in camps for recruits in times of war and national service, the meningococcus lodges in the throats of many susceptible individuals and it is under such conditions that epidemics may occur in the developed countries.

Poliomyelitis

This infection, also known as infantile paralysis, was once a serious cause of death and severe physical handicap in the Western world. In the West vaccination begin during the mid-1950s and poliomyelitis as can be seen from the number of cases per year below:

	1951–5	*1961–5*	*1966–70*	*1976*	*1977*
Britain	4,381	317	24	15	19
USA	37,864	573	52	14	28
Brazil*			11,600	8,652	2,092

*Notified cases only; true figures are much higher.

The disease

In Britain, before vaccination was introduced, the poliovirus was widespread throughout the community. Many children became infected, 99 per cent of these without knowing, and only about one person in a hundred became ill. This made it difficult to understand how the virus spread in the days before we were able to grow the virus so that there were weird and wonderful theories on this subject. In a single school there might be two or three cases but not in the same classroom and perhaps not coming in contact with each other at all. What was not known then was that most of the children in the school had been infected but only a few became ill.

Sometimes the child woke up with a temperature, a headache and the inability to use a limb. Sometimes the respiratory muscles were affected and an 'iron lung' was needed to 'breathe' for the patient. The temperature soon settled and there was sometimes some improvement in the paralysis; however, most patients remained handicapped for the rest of their lives and depended upon the re-education of unaffected muscles to carry out some of the duties of the paralysed muscles.

Avoiding poliomyelitis

The American President Franklin Delano Roosevelt contracted poliomyelitis when he was thirty-nine. He remained handicapped for the rest of his life and, in most photographs of wartime summit meetings, he is sitting while other statesmen are standing. It is thus no coincidence that the American National Foundation for Infantile Paralysis provided the money for the research which first led to the discovery that viruses would grow in tissue culture and which also led to the making of vaccines, not only against polio but also against many other virus diseases.

The virus for the vaccine was grown originally in monkey kidney cells before it was realized what a variety of viruses the normal monkey kidney harboured so that some of those vaccinated against polio in the early days also became immune to most monkey infections!

Killed and live vaccines

As we know by now, a vaccine is basically a suspension of the organisms that normally cause the infection, altered so that they can no longer cause illness.

The simplest way to alter them is to kill them and such vaccines are called 'killed vaccines'. Most bacterial vaccines (i.e. those against typhoid fever, cholera and whooping cough) are of this nature. However, it was found that killed vaccines did not always give a firm immunity and that it was necessary to give at least three injections in most cases. After much experimentation it was found that strains of virus could be grown that caused immunity but did not cause illness when they infected; these were the 'live vaccines'. They had the great advantage that they *did* cause an infection so that they multiply in the body, thus providing a vastly greater amount of virus antigen than if they had been killed. Live vaccine is used to protect against polio, measles and rubella (at least in the West) and one dose is usually enough. (See Figure 6.2.)

Figure 6.2 Killed vaccine versus live vaccine

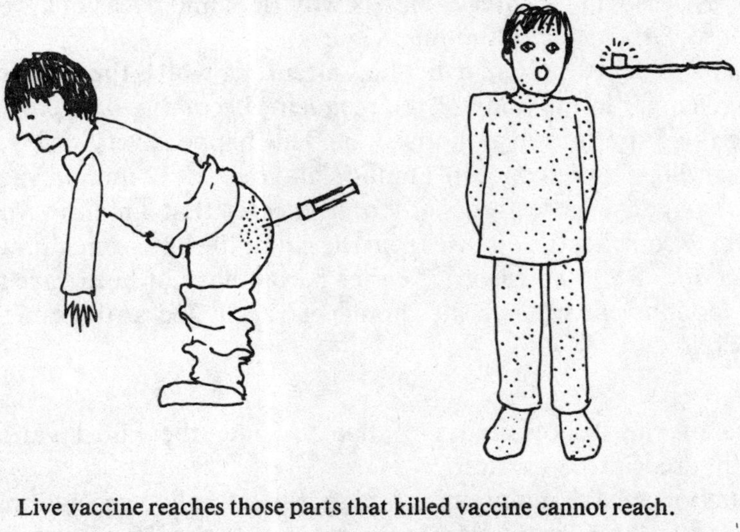

Live vaccine reaches those parts that killed vaccine cannot reach.

The original polio vaccine (the Salk vaccine) was made by killing the virus grown in monkey kidney cells with formaldehyde. What was not realized at that time was that some of the virus was neutralized and was not killed by the formaldehyde; consequently, when the vaccine was diluted, this virus became separated from the formaldehyde and was able to cause infection again. In what was called the Cutter Incident (because of the name of the manufacturing firm involved) in the USA in 1955, there were 204 cases of poliomyelitis and eleven deaths following vaccination with a particular batch of polio vaccine which had not been completely inactivated by formaldehyde. It must have taken great courage for the Americans to carry on with their polio vaccination programme after that!

Today the live vaccine (the Sabin vaccine) is, in the West, used almost exclusively. It uses strains of the three polio viruses that are no longer able to cause infection (or nearly so!). The live vaccine has three drawbacks:

1. It must be kept cold. This can be done in most developed countries but in the Third World, where the vaccine is most needed, it is often impossible to institute a 'cold chain' from the manufacturer to the patient.
2. Interference. The virus in live vaccine infects in the 'natural' way, through the cells of the intestine. If these cells are already infected by a different virus – often the case in countries with poor hygiene – then the polio virus cannot infect. This is why on some occasions we give three doses of vaccine, although it is live.
3. Vaccine-induced poliomyelitis may occur, in which the virus in the vaccine changes in the body of the recipient, becoming dangerous and causing the symptoms of poliomyelitis. This happens very rarely, estimates varying between once in 3 million and once in 12 million vaccinations. A slightly more frequent occurrence is that an *unvaccinated* parent may contract the disease from the child, the latter remaining well and immune. For this reason, if either parent has not been vaccinated against poliomyelitis, he or she should be vaccinated at the same time as the child.

Because of the disadvantages of live vaccine, the killed variety is generally used in the tropics.

The importance of maintaining a high level of polio vaccinations was shown in that half the cases of poliomyelitis in the West occur in the

Netherlands and that all of these particular cases occur in members of a religious sect whose beliefs forbid vaccination.

Tetanus

The name comes form the Greek for 'tightness' and describes the contraction of the muscles, either continuously or in spasms, that occur in this disease. The tetanus bacillus is common in the excreta of horses and some other animals; thus when organic manure is spread on the soil that, too, becomes contaminated. For this reason, during the First World War many of those wounded on the fertile fields of Picardy developed the disease.

This organism resembles the diphtheria bacillus in that it does not invade the body but multiples locally, wherever the wound happens to be, and produces a toxin or poison that spreads throughout the body. The effect of this toxin is to make it too easy for the motor nerves to cause muscles to contract so that muscles that should be quite soft and relaxed become hard and tense. The muscles of the jaw are affected early, hence the popular name 'lockjaw'. As well as producing the permanent constriction of some muscles, the disease induces spasms, like cramp, but more frequent and persistent.

Usually, when we bend our elbow, the biceps muscle contracts to do the work and, to make things easier, the muscles at the back of the arm, needed for straightening it, relax. When tetanus toxin is present there is not this cooperation between groups of muscles and both the 'benders' and the 'straighteners' contract at the same time, causing the painful spasms. (See Figure 6.3.)

Death occurs in about 40 per cent of cases but the death rate is variable and is higher in poorer countries.

Contracting tetanus

The classic case is the elderly allotment owner whose eyes are not as good as they were and who still takes a pride in a well-manured vegetable garden. One day, when using his fork, he puts one of the tines into his foot. After a few days he experiences a little pain in his jaws and difficulty in chewing. His jaw becomes stiffer and stiffer and he may be unable to relax the muscles. Convulsions may follow, involving the spinal muscles, and death from pneumonia or exhaustion may follow.

Tetanus has also followed surgical operations, occasionally in situations where redecoration of operating theatres or adjoining rooms has involved the removal of old plaster from the walls. Such plaster may contain horse hair, added to strengthen it, and the horse hair may have been contaminated with tetanus spores which are still alive after years of dormancy.

Neonatal tetanus

This disease is very rare in Britain but in developing countries it is relatively common. In many places houses are made of a mixture and mud and cow dung and in some cultures cow dung or a mixture of it with other substances is used as a dressing for the umbilical stump. The cow dung contains the tetanus bacillus which multiples in the umbilical stump, produces its toxin and kills the baby. It is no wonder that there are thousands of deaths each year from neonatal tetanus. In the Punjab it is known as the Eight Day Disease because many babies die on the eighth day of life.

Figure 6.3 Tetanus

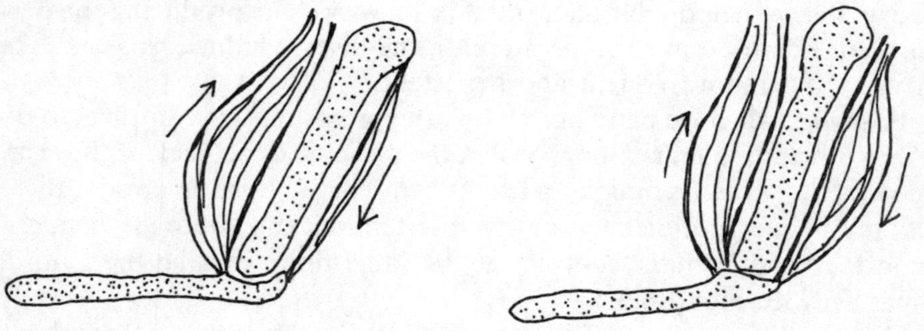

Normal situation. Flexors contract as straighteners relax.

Tetanus present. Both muscle groups contract.

Treating tetanus

The muscle rigidity and spasms may exhaust the patient and, if the respiratory muscles are affected, may prevent him from breathing. Thus treatment includes the administration of curare to the patient; although this drug does not affect the heart, it paralyses all the voluntary muscles, including the respiratory ones. In order to keep the patient breathing an artificial respirator must be used and antibiotics must be administered together with tetanus antiserum. The patient is kept paralysed (but conscious!) for about ten days, by which time the toxin will have been eliminated from the body.

These heroic measures are needed only in very severe cases; in milder cases antitoxin, sedatives and careful nursing in darkened rooms is sufficient.

Avoiding tetanus

Tetanus toxoid is included in the triple vaccine administered in infancy so that most young people will be immune. People with jobs that put them at risk, e.g. agricultural workers, should be revaccinated every five years.

When a person sustains an injury that might have become contaminated by the tetanus bacillus it is sometimes necessary to remove dead tissue surgically and to administer tetanus antiserum. When this used to be produced in horses, there were a great many sensitivy reactions, a few of which proved fatal. Today less reliance is placed on the use of antiserum and, when it is used, the type that is prepared from human serum is preferred.

Rabies

Rabies is a very ancient disease and in the Middle Ages the methods used for its control were quite straightforward—all stray dogs were killed. The disease is caused by a virus shaped like a bullet, which is quite unusual. It is able to infect practically all warmblooded animals.

Mode of infection

The virus is introduced under the skin with the saliva following a bite from an infected animal. The virus passes up along the nerves from the wound to the brain, where it sets up an infection that is invariably fatal.

It also passes to other parts of the body including the salivary glands; this explains how the disease is acquired from infected animals, especially those prone to biting man, e.g. dogs and wolves. Infection from man to man is almost unknown, except for a case when an unfortunate patient developed rabies following a corneal graft taken from a patient who was incubating the disease.

There was also a small outbreak in the North-West Frontier Province of India in young boys following circumcision. The surgeon - barber who carried out the operations was in the habit of smearing his saliva on to the wound at the end of the procedure to promote healing. During the last batch of operations he was, unfortunately, in the late stage of the incubation period for rabies and the virus was present in his saliva.

Rabies is regularly transferred to cattle by the vampire bat in the Americas. However, the role of the bat in spreading the disease has been recently confirmed in Europe, five cases of rabies having followed bites by European bats. This is obviously a matter to be further investigated.

The illness

The illness begins with headache and fever, a sense of foreboding and an itch in the region of a recent bite. Later muscle spasm, delirium and hydrophobia supervene and death takes place within a week of onset.

Hydrophobia is a morbid fear of water and appears as a sort of convulsion of the arms and hands and the swallowing muscles when attempting to drink. It can be brought on by the sight or even the mention of water. A Sudanese doctor once told me that in his country the disease was diagnosed by pouring out a glass of water before the patient. If he did not have a fit, then he was not suffering from rabies! Thus hydrophobia is a symptom of the disease and should not be used as an alternative name for rabies. Hydrophobia does not occur in animals.

Geography and zoology of rabies

The general pattern of the disease is that a dog becomes infected by a wild animal and later bites a human. Known infected animals are:

Europe	Red foxes, dogs, badgers, bats
Americas	Arctic foxes, red foxes, striped skunks, spotted skunks, Mexican freetail bats, vampire bats, cattle
Africa	Dogs, cattle, jackals, wolves, fruit-eating bats
Asia	Dogs, foxes, jackals, wolves, fruit-eating bats

In Europe the animals mainly concerned are red foxes, which are particularly common in northern France. It is always possible that a pet brought into Britain from the Continent has been recently bitten by a red fox; and the Channel Tunnel will need to be made safe against foxes if rabies carriers are to be kept out. Rabies alters the characters of infected animals and affected foxes may come quite close to human habitation, even entering sheds and houses (or even freight cars!).

In the Americas red foxes are also the main carriers, but Mexican freetail bats in Texas and vampire bats in South America also suffer from the disease. The vampire bats pass the disease to cattle, of which least 500,000 head die from rabies each year. However, man is rarely infected in this way; dogs infected by skunks or foxes are the commonest source of human infections.

In Africa there are many types of animal that may become infected, e.g. mongooses, ground squirrels and jackals, but the wild and semi-wild dogs are the greatest menace. These dogs spend their days in the bush and at nights come scavenging into the streets of the towns where they may meet guard dogs whom they infect by biting. Hence, the guard dogs acquire an infection which is a hazard to their human contacts.

In Asia rabies has always been a problem, especially in India among dogs and jackals. In recent years a large outbreak has occurred in China and claimed over 400 lives.

The danger of rabies in Britain

'The man recover'd of the bite; the dog it was that died.' These words of the poet Goldsmith (1730–74) remind us that rabies was fairly common in Britain until about 1903 but, by destroying all affected dogs and quarantining contacts, the disease was eliminated; however, in 1918 it was re-introduced and outbreaks were reported in seventeen counties until it was once more eradicated in 1922. In 1919 a start was made on manufacturing the vaccine in Britain; it was used to vaccinate 144 people bitten by rabid dogs and no cases of the human disease occurred. The quarantining of legally imported dogs has prevented a number of outbreaks, as dogs have developed the disease in the isolation of quarantine kennels. The quarantine period of six months is certainly not too long because dogs have developed the disease after a longer incubation period.

Although there is the danger of human infection to consider, the introduction of rabies into the wild life of Britain would cause us to alter our whole attitude to the countryside; for one thing, it would be necessary to destroy all dogs that were unaccompanied or running free.

Avoiding rabies

It is of vital importance that we keep the infection out of Britain. This has been done so far by careful observations by customs officials and the imposition of heavy fines on those illegally importing animals. These measures have so far proved successful.

Those people who need to work with the virus or in places where rabies occurs or who deal with imported animals must be vaccinated. We have already seen how Pasteur prepared vaccine from the spinal cords of infected rabbits. This vaccine was used for many years (and is still used as a routine measure on patients in India) but is not ideal because nerve tissue, when injected, is very liable to cause severe sensitivity reactions. It may be that in some parts of the world, many people have died from the vaccine rather than the infection. The vaccine is also not very protective and, because of this, up to fourteen injections are needed for vaccination; when the arm and buttock have been used, injections must be given in the abdominal wall—this has given rise to a sort of myth that rabies vaccine must be given intra-abdominally!

It has to be remembered that Pasteur's was a live vaccine and did not necessarily remain harmless. In Brazil in 1960 eighteen patients who had been bitten received rabies vaccine and died from rabies; but it was later shown that only five of the eighteen dogs responsible for the bites had actually suffered from the infection so that up to thirteen patients may have contacted rabies from the vaccine! Since then most kinds of rabies vaccine have been killed vaccine; the virus has been grown in fertile duck eggs and then killed, usually by disinfectants. Most recently a vaccine has been produced from virus grown in tissue culture; it is very pure and very active and preferable to all other kinds. Although there are no cases reported of nurses or doctors catching the infection from patients the greatest of care should be taken in nursing such patients so that staff likely to be dealing with them should be vaccinated. At present about one case of rabies per year occurs in Britain but it has always been contracted abroad.

As we have seen, rabies is one of the few diseases that can be prevented by vaccination *after* infection because of its long incubation period, which is up to a year. Hence, vaccination is used not only to prevent the disease but also to prevent the infection developing into the disease.

What to do if bitten by a dog abroad

If bitten by a dog abroad, find out:

1. If rabies occurs in that country. It is not now present in Britain, Australasia, Japan, Hawaii, Taiwan, the West Indies, Norway and Sweden.
2. If the animal responsible has been kept alive and is available for examination. If the dog is alive and well three weeks later it is most unlikely that it transmitted rabies because rabies is fatal to dog as well as man.

3. If the dog was a stray or a pampered pet. Pampered pets are unlikely to have rabies.
4. If the animal was examined after death and, if so, was rabies diagnosed?
5. If the patient came in contact with the animal's saliva. If not, rabies is unlikely to develop.

If the answers to these points suggest that it is *not unlikely* that the patient has suffered the risk of rabies infection, he should receive the vaccine as soon as possible.

Because the earlier vaccines were unpleasant and inefficient, we have tended not to vaccinate in doubtful situations. The tissue culture vaccine is without side effects and very efficient so that we now tend to vaccinate in all situations except when the risk of infection is very remote.

The slow viruses

These are responsible for an interesting group of diseases, at least one, Bovine Spongiform Encephalitis (BSE), being of topical interest. There are two types of organism responsible for slow virus infections: conventional viruses and unconventional agents.

Diseases caused by conventional viruses

The measles virus is an example of a disease caused by a conventional virus and, in a few cases of measles, the virus remains in the body after infection. Many years later this may cause severe and often fatal encephalitis; while uncommon, it is serious when it does occur. The term 'slow' refers to the long incubation period of all these diseases. The condition caused by the measles virus is known as Subacute Sclerosing Panencephalitis (SSPE); a similar condition known as Progressive Multifocal Leucoencephalopathy (PML) may be caused by several viruses, including those known as JC, SV40 (a virus infecting monkeys) and BK.

Two sheep infections Visna and Maedi are also caused by conventional viruses as is Aleutian Mink Disease (AM), which was first noticed in a blue-grey mutation of ranch mink in 1941. It was demonstrated to be infectious following the use of home-made distemper vaccine, which was made by boiling the spleen of a distemper infected mink in dilute formalin. When the spleen came from a mink already also infected with AM disease, thousands of those inoculated developed the disease.

Diseases caused by unconventional agents

These organisms are unique in that they are still infectious after boiling for three hours and after autoclaving at 110°C for thirty minutes. They are also very resistant to disinfectants and irradiation. These strange properties are believed to be due to the fact that they lack a protein coat which conventional viruses possess and which facilitates their attachment to host cells. This coat is heat sensitive so that conventional viruses are destroyed easily by heat. The lack of a protein coat may go some way to explaining the slow progress made by the agent from cell to cell and hence the long incubation period of the disease.

The following diseases are caused by unconventional agents:

Scrapie
Bovine Spongiform Encephalitis (BSE)
Transmissible Mink Encephalopathy (TME)
Kuru
Creuzfeldt-Jakob Disease (CJD)

Some of these are discussed below.

Scrapie

Scrapie is a fatal disease of sheep known in Western Europe for over 200 years. It can be transmitted to healthy sheep and has an incubation period of from one to over five years. The disease has also been transmitted to mice. It is infectious between sheep and is present in the body fluids apart from the central nervous system.

Bovine spongiform encephalitis

Bovine Spongiform Encephalitis (BSE or 'Mad Cow Disease') is scrapie in cattle. It is not likely to cause human infection, since we have been eating scrapie-infected mutton for 200 years. The name describes the condition: the brain is infected and, where cells are killed, small holes appear, giving the brain the appearance of a sponge under the microscope. It is an important disease for farmers but would seem to have little public health significance.

Kuru and Creuzfeldt-Jakob disease

Kuru – Eating people is wrong and can seriously injure your health. In 1955 it was found that the principal cause of death among the Fore people of New Guinea – about 30,000 strong – was a condition called 'kuru' (meaning 'I fall about'). This was a slow encephalitis: the patient became unsteady, had difficulty in walking, and eventually took to his bed and died. It was shown that the disease was transmissable and could be passed to chimpanzees and other primates (but not mice).

In the 1950s 90 per cent of adult deaths among the Fore people was due to Kuru. Before 1956 these people practised cannibalism, which was at first an act of hostility towards killed and captured enemies but later became part of the funeral ceremonies for relatives. Women and young children partook of the human flesh and they were more often affected than the men. Cannabilism was discontinued about 1956 and the incidence of kuru has since diminished, although the appearance of sporadic cases indicated an incubation period in excess of twenty-five years.

Creuzfeldt-Jakob Disease (CJD) is a rare disease that was originally believed to be degenerative in nature – the brain was wearing out at an earlier age than usual. The disease affects men and women who are mainly in their sixties and starts with attacks of depression and confusion, leading on to difficulties in walking, dementia and death usually within a year. The condition can be transmitted to many laboratory animals and has been accidentally transmitted from patient to patient. In one instance a man developed CJD after a corneal transplant, the donor dying of the disease two years later. The second case involved the use of electrodes implanted in the brain; they had been previously used on a CJD patient.

Any suggestion that CJD is caused by eating scrapie-contaminated mutton is contradicted by the fact that the disease occurs in lifelong vegetarians.

It would be tempting to believe that kuru had arisen from an incident when a missionary with incipient CJD had gone to New Guinea to preach the Gospel. Unfortunately he ended up on the menu of a group of Fore people. In this way his influence was greater and longer lasting than if he had confined himself to preaching. Unfortunately there is no evidence to support this theory.

SEVEN

Sexually Acquired Infections

Until about the 1940s there were only two commonly recognized diseases known to be spread by sexual intercourse: syphilis and gonorrhoea. When antibiotics appeared on the scene it was found that the organisms causing these diseases were very sensitive and it seemed for a while as if venereologists would soon become redundant!

However, since then a number of other conditions have emerged to take the places of these earlier diseases which, though less common, are still with us. For instance, between 1960 and 1975 there were about 20,000 new cases of syphilis in the USA each year. New cases in Britain for syphilis have been:

Year	*Number of cases*
1946	20,000
1979	4,385
1981	4,211
1983	3,727
1984	3,307

Fortunately, syphilis has generally speaking remained sensitive to common antibiotics—as is also the case with gonorrhoea.

The new sexually acquired diseases include hepatitis B, chlamydial infection, genital herpes and, more recently, AIDS. The organisms capable of causing these diseases do so because they are extremely delicate ones and are killed easily by cold and dryness. Thus very close—indeed, intimate—contact is necessary for them to pass from one person to another and survive so that the only ways in which they can spread are through actual sexual intercourse—heterosexual or homosexual—and other intimate pastimes such as kissing.

Sexually acquired diseases used to be known as venereal diseases. The word 'venereal' is a hangover from the days when love and sex were coincident, being derived from Venus, the goddess of Love.

Syphilis

This disease was given its name following the publication of a poem by Fracostorius, a Venetian poet and scientist, in 1530. The poem was a summary of what was then known of the disease and, according to the poem, the first man to contract it was a swineherd called Syphilos.

The disease first arrived in Europe about 1493 following the return of Columbus from the island of Haiti and many people believe that it originated in America. Gabriel Fallopius, after whom the Fallopian tubes were named, said about this time: 'For Columbus brought back his vessels laden with the French disease. There the disease is mild, like the Itch amongst us, but transplanted hither it has become so fierce and unmerciful, as to infect and corrupt the head, eyes, nose, palate, skin, flesh, bones, ligaments and at last the whole bowels'. Indeed, when it first appeared in Europe it was a very acute disease, running its course very rapidly and frequently causing death in quite a short time. Such behaviour is typical of an infection introduced into a community which has never known it before.

The Europeans had difficulty in agreeing to a name for this new disease before the name syphilis became established. The Spaniards called it the disease of Espanola, the Italians called it the French disease, the French called it the Italian disease, the English called it the French pox, the Russians called it the Polish disease, for the Turks it was the French disease and for Indians and Japanese it was the Portuguese disease.

The moralists seized upon the disease as being a manifestation of the wrath of God on sinful people—compare some present attitudes to AIDS—especially in view of the way it was contracted, although a few unusual 'causes' were quoted, including bestiality and the eating of lizards. Even until recent times the disease has been used like a moral hammer. Victorian, and later, novels refer to it as a 'foul disease', usually contracted by the villain. Whenever a hero contracts it, he is usually a surgeon who cuts himself when operating on an infected case; he then gives up all hope of marrying and devotes himself to his work, for fear of infecting his wife and children—although even a surgeon should be aware of the fact that even the untreated disease is no longer infectious after about four years.

Cardinal Wolsley was accused of giving Henry VIII syphilis by whispering in his ear but this must have been unique in the history of the transmission of the disease!

The illness

When syphilis is untreated today, it runs a much slower course than it did when it first reached Europe. It usually passes, through three stages:

1. *The primary stage of infection*

The primary stage is nearly always by sexual intercourse, although it may rarely come about through kissing or, more rarely, by cuts acquired at post-mortems or during surgical operations. The first sign, which appears about three weeks after infection, is a painless ulcer on the penis in the male and, in the female, an ulcer within the vagina, which is rarely observed by the patient.

Because the male sexual organ is so much more easily available for inspection a man is far more likely to notice his infection—called a chancre—than a woman. At this stage it is possible to diagnose the condition from the history, the appearance of the chancre and by putting on the ulcer a little saline, which can be looked at with a micrcoscope. In positive cases large numbers of delicate spiral organisms may be seen. These organisms cause the disease, which is known as *Spirochoeta pallida*—the pale spirochoete. It resembles a tiny spring that has been pulled out to form a 'corkscrew'.

It is very difficult to stain and is usually looked for using a darkground microscope, in which the matter on the slide is illuminated from the side and not from below. By this procedure the spirochoete, and any other organisms present, appear as bright objects on a black background. The stage of the chancre is the first stage of syphilis.

2. *The secondary stage of infection*

If syphilis in the primary stage is not treated, after a while there will be a sufficient number of spirochoetes to invade the blood and thence the whole body. There then occurs the secondary stage, which is very much like the 'rash' stage in measles, chickenpox, etc. The skin rash and ulcers that appear on the palate are rich with spirochoetes and at this stage the patient is highly infectious. The skin rash and ulcers occur about two to eight weeks after the first ulcer on the genitalia appears.

3. *The tertiary stage of infection*
If the secondary stage is not treated the patient may appear to recover and may remain well for years; the tertiary stage may not appear until 5 or 10 years later (or even longer). However, the spirochoetes will have caused damage throughout the body. The three main systems damaged are the spinal cord, the brain and the large blood vessels.
a. *Tabes dorsalis.* This condition results from damage to those nerves in the spinal cord which give us position sense. If we stand with our eyes closed we do not usually fall over because sense organs in the skin of the feet are constantly passing messages up to the spinal cord which can be translated into warnings that we are leaning too far one way or the other; immediately messages pass to the muscles to counteract this tendency. This happens many times a second and in this way we keep—when sober—more or less vertical. If a patient who is suffering from tabes and whose special nerve fibres have been damaged, closes his eyes, he tends to keel over; early sign of this is a tendency to bang his head on the washbasin tap when washing his face. He also tends to walk with a peculiar high-stepping gait. Tabes also results in bladder disturbances and impotence.
b. *General Paralysis of the Insane.* GPI begins with the patient developing delusions, usually of grandeur. Out of the blue he will offer to buy Buckingham Palace or complain that the Prime Minister is plotting against him. His delusions slowly 'burn out' and he becomes weaker and weaker, finally becoming paralysed and then dying.
c. *Aortic aneurysm.* The spirochoetes damage the wall of this great artery until it cannot withstand the internal pressure and it begins to 'balloon' like a car inner tube through a hole in the outer case of the tyre. Then what usually happens is that in the vessel bursts with fatal results. (See Figure 7.1.) (Most cases of aneurysm occurring today are due to other causes.)

All these late complications of syphilis are rare today because the primary infection is usually treated promptly and effectively.

Treatment and prevention of syphilis

The spirochoete of syphilis is very sensitive to penicillin and, if given during either of the first two stages of infection, the patient is cured. In the third stage much damage will have been done to various tissues and this cannot be reversed; nevertheless, penicillin may still be useful even in this stage. At one time it was believed that high fever was beneficial for patients suffering from GPI and for this reason they were deliberately injected with malarial parasites to give them the infection and hence a raised body temperature. Penicillin has made this mode of treatment obsolete.

Figure 7.1 Aneurysm of the aorta

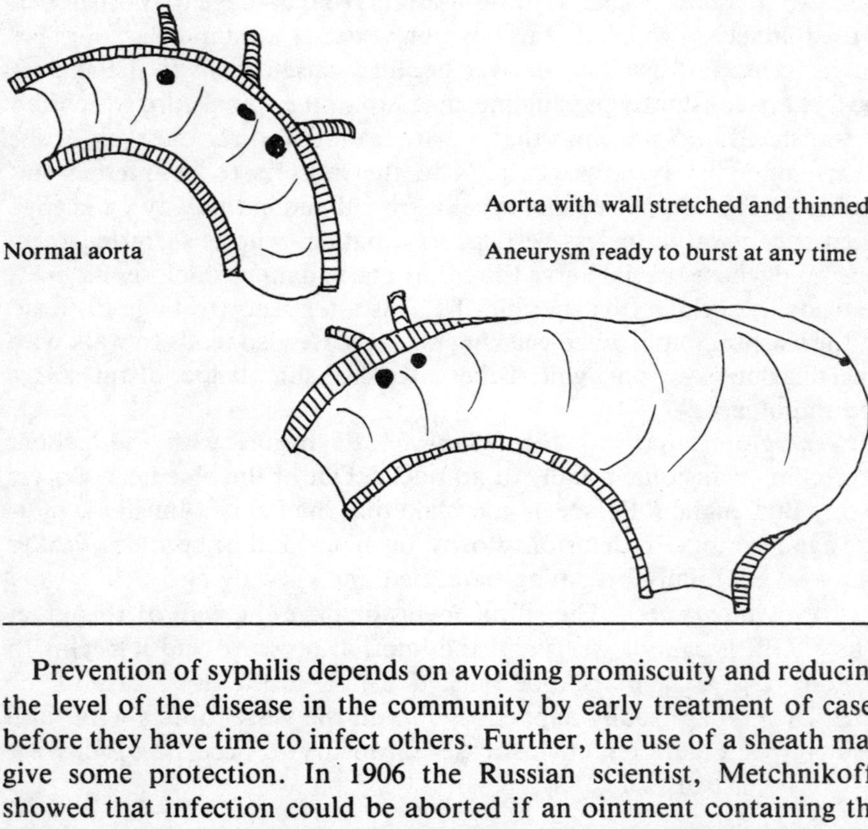

Prevention of syphilis depends on avoiding promiscuity and reducing the level of the disease in the community by early treatment of cases before they have time to infect others. Further, the use of a sheath may give some protection. In 1906 the Russian scientist, Metchnikoff, showed that infection could be aborted if an ointment containing the mercury salt calomel were applied to the infected parts within a few hours. In 1910 he received a Nobel prize; was there a connection?

Gonorrhoea

For many years this disease was the constant companion of syphilis. When I was a student they were practically the only venereal diseases recognized and were constantly seen together.

In the eighteenth century the celebrated experimental physician, John Hunter, deliberately injected pus from a case of gonorrhoea into his skin; he believed that gonorrhoea and syphilis were caused by the same organism, syphilis following a skin infection and gonorrhoea following infection of mucous membranes; unfortunately, the patient from whom the pus came really had syphilis *and* gonorrhoea. Hunter developed syphilis and probably died from it. Even today, when the treatment of gonorrhoea is usually very short and simple, it has to be borne in mind that the patient may be incubating syphilis while suffering from gonorrhoea.

The name of the disease means 'flow of seed'; the early physicians did not have microscopes and mistook the purulent discharge for a flow of semen. The bacterium that causes the disease was named after the disease—the gonococcus, *Neisseria gonorrhoeae*, is a close relation of the common cause of meningitis, *Neisseria meningitidis*.

As with other organisms that cause venereal diseases, the gonococcus is a very delicate organism and it will not survive the ordeal of being carried about on a swab at room temperature for any length of time.

As we have seen, not only does the organism cause venereal disease but it used to cause about a quarter of the blindness in the world through congenital infection. Even today gonorrhoea is a very prevalent disease. The number of reported cases in the USA rose from 300,000 cases in 1965 to 1,000,000 in 1975 and the real numbers were probably about three times as great. Some recent figures for gonorrhoea in Britain are:

Year	*Number of cases*
1979	61,616
1980	60,850
1982	50,778
1984	53,080

Gonorrhoea is a disease with a short incubation period—a few days—and is usually rapidly cured by antibiotics. This means that a patient may be back to the clinic with another infection within six weeks of his previous treatment and some individuals have been known to experience over twenty infections.

The illness

The gonococcus infects the membrane lining the urethra (the tube through which urine flows from the bladder) and stimulates the formation of pus. This results in a discharge and stained films of this discharge show large numbers of gonococci.

When an infected man has sexual intercourse with an uninfected woman, the end of the penis comes into contact with the cervix (the neck of the womb) and may infect it. The organisms causing gonorrhoea multiply there and if the woman later has intercourse with an uninfected man, he is likely to contract a urethral infection from this site. If the infection is treated early with antibiotics the organism is readily killed and the patient recovers completely. If untreated, the organism tends to move up the genital tract. In the man it moves to the prostate and can begin a longstanding infection that may cause the urethra to constrict, damming back the urine and damaging the kidneys. In former days a VD clinic would have on its books several elderly male patients who came solely for the passage of 'bougies' which enlarged the constriction and which allowed a fairly free flow of urine until their next visit. (See Figure 7.2.)

Figure 7.2 Gonorrhoea in the male

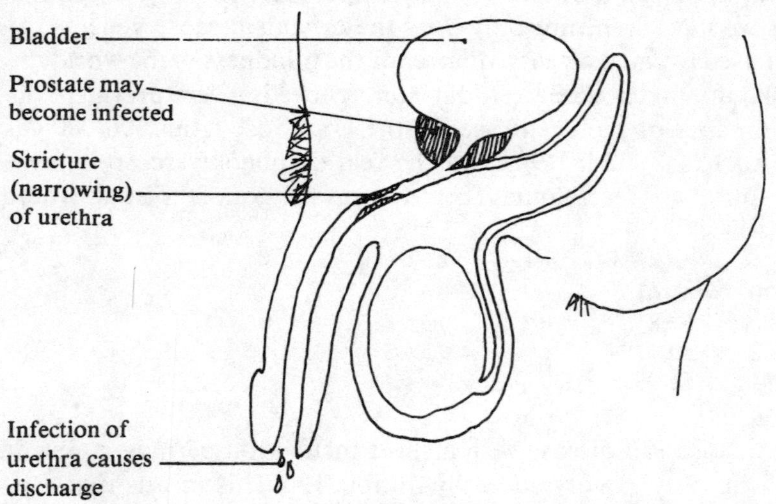

In women the organism moves upwards and, although the uterus is not infected because of its habit of shedding its lining every month, the organism may 'jump the gap' and cause infection of the Fallopian tubes. This condition ('hot tubes') causes severe chronic infection and used to be a common cause of sterility because it resulted in the tubes becoming blocked. As with syphilis, the female anatomy makes it difficult for a woman to know if she has been infected and many women have passed the disease on quite innocently. (See Figure 7.3.)

Figure 7.3 Gonorrhoea in the female

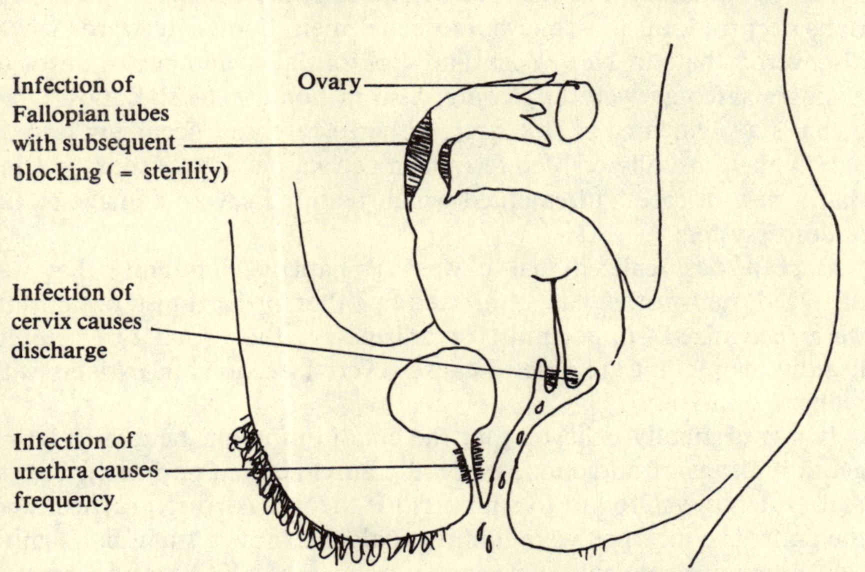

Acquired Immune Deficiency Syndrome (AIDS)

As we have seen, toward the end of the fifteenth century a new disease, later called syphilis, appeared in the West; hitherto unknown, it was spread by sexual intercourse and untreatable. About five centuries later a similar disease emerged; it was eventually to be called Acquired Immune Deficiency Syndrome and is better known to most people as AIDS.

It is important to remember that AIDS is the last stage of infection by the virus now known as the Human Immunodeficiency Virus (HIV). It was originally believed that only 10 per cent to 16 per cent of patients infected with the virus responsible would develop the disease AIDS. However, as groups of patients are followed up over longer periods, more and more of their number progress from the symptomless infection to full-blown AIDS. It now seems that most or even all of those infected who live long enough will develop and die from the disease known as AIDS.

The emergence of AIDS

There is a small parasite known as *Pneumocystis carinii* which rarely causes illness in healthy people, although it may do so in patients with damaged immunity. In June 1981 a number of these formerly rare infections occurred, all in young homosexual men. Soon afterwards it was discovered that, in New York and California, a number of cases of Kaposi's sarcoma were appearing, also in homosexuals. Kaposi's sarcoma is a pigmented skin cancer, hitherto rare and occurring only in elderly men, usually of Mediterranean extraction. It was soon realized that a new disease had emerged which featured severe damage to the immune system.

Once it was realized that it was the patients' immunity that was damaged, many other cases, infected by other 'opportunist' organisms, were recognized – opportunist organisms are those that rarely infect healthy people but are able to cause severe infections in patients with reduced immunity.

It was originally believed that the condition might be due to indulgence in drugs of addiction, especially amyl nitrite ('poppers'), but no real evidence was found to support this theory. At first practically all the patients concerned were homosexuals, but now a small but significant number of patients suffering from haemophilia began to develop the condition, together with drug addicts who used the intravenous route and who tended to share syringes with their colleagues. This at once suggested that the condition was a bloodborne infection and, with infinitely more resources than it possessed in the early days of syphilis, medical science set out to find the cause and, if possible, either a cure or a method of prevention.

The virus

The 'AIDS virus' belongs to a large group known as 'retroviruses', which includes some capable of causing malignant disease. Its discovery illustrates the keen rivalry that exists between many scientists today.

Workers in Paris isolated, in early 1983, a virus from a homosexual man with enlarged lymph glands – a condition which may occur after HIV infection but before the development of full-blown AIDS – but it was only with great difficulty that this virus was persuaded to grow in the laboratory.

In the USA a different virus had been isolated and the Americans believed that it was the cause of AIDS. A sample of this virus (known simply as HTLV) was sent to Paris but the French found it was very different from the one they had isolated, now known as LAV. An account of the isolation of the French virus from cases of AIDS was sent to an eminent American scientific journal but its author was first persuaded by the Americans to describe their virus as 'a member of the human T-cell leukaemia virus (HTLV) family', i.e. to state, under pressure, that the French virus *was* related to the American candidate. This journal also contained at the same time three American articles describing their HTLV virus as the cause of AIDS and the French article was overlooked.

The French had twice sent samples of their virus to the American laboratory but the first sample was said to have died on the way. In April 1984 the Americans claimed to have discovered 'a new variant' of the HTLV virus which they called HTLV-3. An American Secretary of the Department of Health announced that 'the probable cause of AIDS has been found – a variant of a known human cancer virus, called HTLV-3'. Credit, she added, should go to the American scientist who directed the research that produced this discovery. (The AIDS virus is certainly *not* a cancer virus as are the HTLV-1 and 2 viruses.)

There appear to be only three indicators and rewards of human success: sex, money and credit. We can discount the first as being a private matter but the other two are just as much appreciated by medical researchers as by other members of the community.

As far as credit is concerned, there is great jealousy in scientific circles about priority of publication; if a scientist were to forecast the end of the world with some confidence he might well be remembered to the end of time, no matter how short a period that might be; if an equally convincing forecast were to be made by an equally confident worker but published a day later, the latter would be practically ignored. Thus, although the virus that caused AIDS appeared to have been discovered in France, it seemed that the credit might go to the USA although its discovery came a year later.

As far as the financial side was concerned, money is important to scientists as it is to lesser men. The money concerned may not be for private use but perhaps to finance laboratory expansion, staff increases or travel to other centres of learning. It is an unusual catastrophe that does not line the pockets of some person or institution and the demand for blood tests for the diagnosis of AIDS would be worth many millions of pounds. American lawyers at once applied for a patent on the use of the American 'AIDS virus' which would be the basis of such tests and, if the French had discovered the virus the previous year, this was manifestly unfair.

One very significant comment was made by Nature herself on these affairs. As we shall see later, the AIDS virus – now called the Human

Immunodeficiency Virus (HIV) because it is not related to the human cancer viruses – is very labile; this means that the chemicals on its surface are constantly changing, as in the case of the influenza virus, but much faster. Thus strains isolated at different times or from different locations may be quite different from each other. The patient from whom the French virus (LAV) had been isolated had not been to the USA since 1979, several years before the isolation of the American 'HTLV' virus. However, in 1985 twelve different strains of 'AIDS' viruses from various sources were carefully analysed together with five isolated from a single location, New York. The researchers found that all the isolates were different – even those isolated at about the same time from New York – *except the French (LAV) and the American (HTLV-3)*, which appeared identical. This strongly suggested that the Americans might have derived, no doubt by accident, their strain of the 'AIDS virus' from the strain they received from France in 1983.

A fuller account of the not entirely creditable proceedings and of the strange way in which the affair was concluded is given in *The Search for the Virus* by Steve Connor and Sharon Kingman (Penguin Books 1988).

How AIDS infection causes illness

When a crime occurs in a civilized community it is usual for the police to apprehend the criminal and restrain him from further wrongdoing. If a gang of criminals 'neutralize' the police force, then all sorts of petty thieves, who would not normally disturb the peace, would be able to go on the rampage with impunity. (See Figure 7.4 and 7.5.)

The latter is what happens in AIDS. After the patient has become infected with HIV, the virus invades and multiplies in certain white cells

Figure 7.4 T-cells preserve immunity and repel opportunist organisms

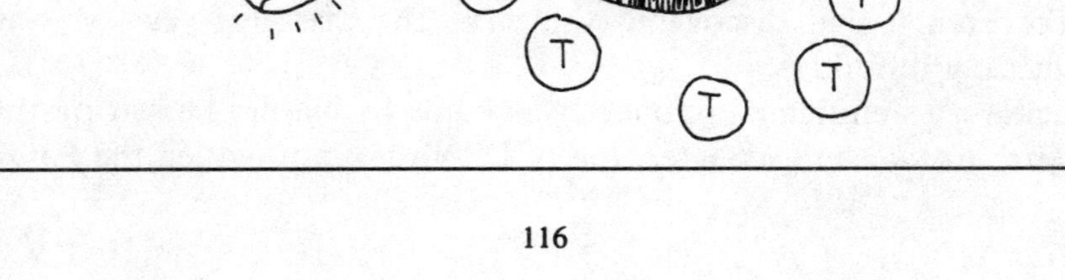

which are essential for efficient immunity and are known as 'helper T-cells'. The virus nucleic acid finds its way into the chromosomes of these white cells and becomes part of the cell nucleus.

After a variable time – usually measured in years – the virus begins to kill these white cells and the dramatic fall in their number is reflected by a deterioration in the patient's immunity and the ease with which

Figure 7.5 H.I.V. destroys T-cells and lets in opportunists

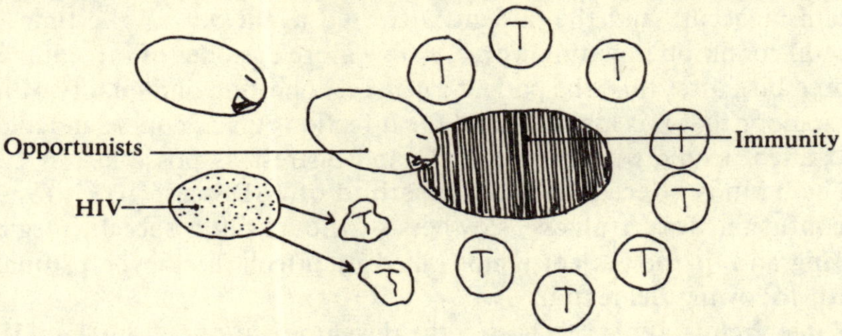

'opportunist' organisms – the petty criminals of infection – are able to cause severe and eventually fatal infection. Thus there are two important points. The first is that full-blown AIDS was originally believed to occur in only a proportion of those infected with HIV and only after a long incubation period; at present it is believed that 10 per cent to 15 per cent of those infected will contract the illness but our knowledge of the infection is too short for us to be sure that, in time, all those infected will not be eventually affected.

The other point is that HIV itself *does not kill*, but opens the door to the assassain; death is caused by a variety of opportunist infections. The opportunistic infective agents include *Pneumocystis carinii*, Kaposi's sarcoma (which appears to be an infective tumour), cytomegalovirus, the herpes virus, fungi such as those causing thrush and tubercle bacilli, and, among many others, bacteria, parasites and fungi that have little effect on normal persons.

The course of AIDS

The diagnosis of AIDS is not usually difficult because it occurs mainly in patients of a certain type – homosexual men, intravenous drug addicts, haemophiliacs or sexual contacts of one of these groups – so that the doctor should suspect the diagnosis at once, especially if the patient has a cough and shortness of breath or evidence of Kaposi's sarcoma. A test for antibodies to HIV should be made and, if negative, repeated monthly for at least three months.

Most patients developing AIDS die within three years, if not sooner: those whose onset of disease was signalled by Kaposi's sarcoma live for an average of about two years and those with pneumonia at the onset die after about a year. The progress of the disease is usually typical. The original infection may be treated with suitable antibiotics and the patient may then remain well for a few months. Soon infection by a different organism occurs and the patient is treated again but all the time his general condition is getting worse. A few more episodes of infection are treated but, after this, the patient's general condition and quality of life are so poor that it is kindest to let the infection run its course and allow the patient to die with as little pain and distress as possible.

The brain is affected in about one third of AIDS cases. This results in confusion, forgetfulness, slowness of thought and speech, illegible writing and, if the patient is not killed by infection elsewhere, finally death following dementia.

Three factors appear to hasten the development of full-blown AIDS in infected persons. The acquisition of further sexually spread diseases, such as gonorrhoea appears to reduce the incubation period in men. In women who are merely infected and have no symptoms pregnancy appears to hasten the onset of the disease (and about 50 per cent of babies born to infected mothers are themselves infected) and HIV infection in these babies tends to lead to AIDS more often and more quickly than in adults.

Who contracts AIDS?

In the USA the early victims were active homosexuals and that situation still prevails in most western countries. In Britain, for example, by May 1990 out of a total of 2898 cases of fully developed AIDS that had occurred since the beginning of the outbreak, 85 per cent were male homosexuals, 2.3 per cent were male intravenous drug abusers, 0.7 per cent were female drug abusers, 1.4 per cent were male homosexual drug abusers, 6.2 per cent were haemophiliacs, 1.7 per cent had received blood transfusions (mostly abroad), 5.1 per cent were heterosexuals (4 per cent contracted abroad, 0.5 per cent contracted in Britain and 0.8 per cent contacts) and 0.8 per cent were children born to HIV-infected mothers. It is interesting to note that practically all British cases of AIDS among intravenous drug abusers occurred in Edinburgh where 40 per cent of drug addicts are HIV positive (infection contracted by use of contaminated syringes); as more females tend to become infected by this route than by any other, the incidence of infected babies born to infected mothers in Scotland is about forty times higher than that in the rest of Britain. The sharing of syringes is still a commoner way for women to become infected in the West than by heterosexual activities with infected men.

How HIV infection is spread

As we have seen, the HIV infects helper T-cells, cells that are present in the blood and also in semen. Very few virus particles are free in the fluid part of blood or semen, but each infected T-cell contains thousands. This seems to explain why HIV infection is spread mainly through semen – homosexual and heterosexual intercourse – and through blood – contaminated syringes, Factor 8 for haemophiliacs, by blood transfusion (no longer a major cause in western countries where each unit of blood is checked for antibody) and, rarely, by 'needle-stick' accidents in hospitals.

One (African) worker has suggested that HIV infection is frequently the result of abnormal sex; abnormal in amount, as with some prostitutes, or abnormal in type, as in homosexual intercourse (if, indeed, the second most popular form of sex can be described as abnormal!) Homosexuals have tended to be far more profligate and less discriminatory with their favours than heterosexuals (although the menace of AIDS has lately diminished this tendency) and this probably accounts for the early rapid spread of the infection among homosexuals, especially in the developed world. Oddly enough, following heterosexual intercourse, women are more likely to become infected by infected men than the other way round.

Laboratory diagnosis of AIDS

There was just as much rivalry in the search for a test for HIV infection – it is *not* AIDS at this stage – as there was to discover the virus. A new class of tests for antibody in infections had been developed over the previous fifteen years or so, known as ELISA tests (the full name probably manipulated so as to give an attractive acronym). These tests depend on the fact that antigen (in this case virus) can be fixed to plastic.

The test is carried out using either tubes, plates with wells or spheres of plastic to which have been attached HIV. The patient's blood serum is placed in the well or tube, allowed to incubate for a while and then washed away. If there was any antibody to HIV in the serum, this will have become firmly fixed to the virus and hence to the tube – *it will not wash away*. The antibody is then detected by adding a substance carrying an enzyme that is capable of attaching itself to the trapped antibody. It is now only necessary to add a solution of the chemical that the enzyme is capable of breaking down to detect the presence of antibody by a change of colour. (See Figure 7.6.)

Figure 7.6 The ELISA test for antibody

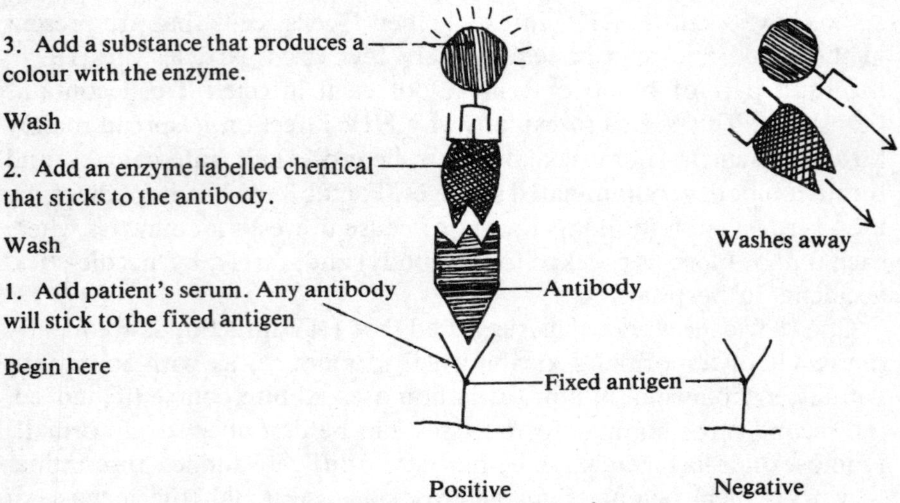

This test is not 100 per cent accurate and tends to give false positives – especially in people who have or have had multiple infections from various other organisms. For this reason a slightly modified test, known as the 'competitive ELISA test', is used in Britain.

Random testing for HIV infection

The expected number of positive reactions among blood donors, i.e. ordinary members of the public, is very low. This means that the numbers of positive results subjects giving a false negative test will be small enough to ignore. On the other hand, quite a few who are really negative may give false positive results; these are the results that will need to be checked by repeating the test and by using more refined tests that are too complicated for routine use.

If widespread random testing were carried out the false positive would be embarrassing. Suppose a test identifies correctly 99 per cent of the positive cases and 99 per cent of the negative cases. Suppose, again, we test (to simplify the mathematics) 1,000,020 members of the public, of whom about twenty people per million are genuinely positive. As the test picks up 99 per cent of the real positives, all twenty in our population would be identified. However, of those who were not positive the test would wrongly label 1 per cent, i.e. 10,000 persons, as positive. Thus the gross results of the exercise would be 10,020 positive tests and the real work would begin in deciding how many and which were really positive!

Antibody does not appear in infected patients until from six weeks to six months after infection. Hence, there is a remote risk in blood transfusion practice that a donation may be made by a person who has been recently infected but who has not yet produced antibody. At this stage there may be antigen, i.e. virus, in his blood and tests for detecting virus have been devised. These tests may be useful for the diagnosis of AIDS in *individuals* during the early stages of infection but, so far, they have not produced extra positive tests when used for screening blood donations.

AIDS in Africa

One of the smaller groups of people in the West who developed AIDS consisted of people with links with Africa. Black people from Africa were found in 1983 to be suffering from the disease although they had been in Europe for sometimes as long as three years, while in 1977 a Danish woman surgeon had died from what was almost certainly AIDS in Zaire where she had lived and worked since 1972. In Zambia it was noticed in the early 1980s that Kaposi's sarcoma was occurring in young men who were subsequently dying; formerly it had occurred in old men who they had survived, even without treatment.

When testing for antibody became available a number of surveys were carried out, with dramatic results. One such survey indicated that over 60 per cent of healthy children in a district of Uganda had antibodies to AIDS. Such results gave rise to suspicions about the ELISA test that was being used. When a more efficient test—the 'competitive ELISA test' used in Britain from the beginning—was used together with more complicated confimatory tests, it was found that the numbers of subjects positive were not as great as was first believed. The presence of large numbers of potentially infectious agents in the environment results in a great variety of different antibodies in the blood of the local people and these react in the test, giving false positive results.

However, AIDS is common in Africa and never more so than along the main highways where the 'bar girls' entertain the truck drivers at their overnight stopping places. About 70 per cent of the 'bar girls' were found to have antibody – this time using a reliable test – as were 17 per cent of mothers attending an immunization clinic with their children, of whom 1 per cent were positive. When the truck drivers were tested, about 30 per cent were infected; it appeared that many had had over fifty sexual partners during their relatively short lives – although the type of sex was normal, the numbers were not!

AIDS in Africa appears to be spread mainly by heterosexual intercourse so that the incidences in men and women are practically identical. It is also possible that the re-use of imperfectly sterilized syringes and needles plays a part in the spread of the infection and this, too, would result in a one-to-one sex ratio.

The symptoms of AIDS are caused by opportunist organisms so that we would expect to find that AIDS sufferers become infected by those opportunists most prevalent in the part of the world where they live; thus, in Africa intestinal infections are common and the occurrence of diarrhoea and weight loss in African AIDS patients has given the name 'slim disease' to the condition. There is no doubt that the problem of AIDS in Africa and other parts of the Third World is going to be far more serious than in the West.

When the African connection with AIDS was discovered and when it was found that Americans with connections with Haiti were liable to contract the disease, it was concluded that another virus infection had come out of Africa. However, in the last year or so the prehistory of AIDS has needed to be rewritten from time to time. Examination of stored blood from Africans did not, at first, reveal the HIV antibody in any specimens taken earlier than the late 1970s. However, Norwegian doctors showed, by examining stored serum, that a family of three, mother, father and daughter, had all died of AIDS in 1976 in Norway and that the mother and father had developed the early symptoms of AIDS as early as 1966–7. More recently, antibody to the virus has been demonstrated in stored blood taken from an African in Zaire in 1959, and tissue specimens taken post mortem from a twenty-five year old seaman who died of pneumonia in the same year in Manchester, England, have been shown to contain segments of nucleic acid identical with those in the AIDS virus. He was at sea during 1955–7, but none of his ports of call have been revealed. The AIDS virus must have been about for a long time before AIDS was recognized as an infection in 1981. The arrival of syphilis in Europe may well have been due to its importation by the contemporaries of Colombus from America where it was rife; no such new found land can be held responsible for the emergence of AIDS.

The genesis of AIDS, that is, its origin as a virus, is as obscure as its spread. Several related viruses have been discovered in sheep, goats, cattle, horses and monkeys. The viruses infecting the latter—simian immunodeficiency viruses (SAIDS)—resemble HIV more closely than the others. The relationships between viruses are estimated by determining the similarity of the nucleic acid sequences in their genes. A SAID affecting the monkey known as the sooty mangabey closely resembles the virus known as HIV2, which causes illness in humans in parts of West Africa; however, the resemblances of these viruses to HIV1 (as we have to call the immunodeficiency virus responsible for AIDS world wide) is not great; as with other SAIDS it is only about 55 per cent. More recently, though, a virus has been isolated from a chimpanzee which has up to an 84 per cent resemblance. This suggests that the AIDS virus might have developed from a chimpanzee virus but, so far, only one specimen of the latter has been isolated and that from a captive animal; it is not impossible that the virus might have been acquired from human sources. Obviously more detective work is necessary.

One less likely theory is that the virus has been present for a long time in a closed community which has fairly recently opened up and that modern conditions, such as the widespread use of syringes and needles, have facilitated the spread.

Prevention and treatment of HIV infection and AIDS

For specific prevention a vaccine is needed but this will prove difficult to perfect because:

1. The surface of the virus is constantly changing. This means that if a given strain is used to make a vaccine protection will be against that strain only; as we have seen, even from one location at about the same time, several different strains may be expected. When we discuss the influenza virus we shall find that it undergoes a similar antigenic change, but in this case it is measured over years and a vaccine made from the current strain would be likely to be effective for ten years or so.
2. There is no real evidence that the antibody induced by vaccination would protect against infection. Antibody is present in the blood of all cases of HIV infection except for some cases of terminal AIDS but it does not protect from progressive illness. There are other infections—including that caused by the herpes simplex virus, for instance—where

the virus can re-infect in the presence of antibody in the blood.
3. No small laboratory animals are susceptible to the infection so that any experimental work must be carried out on man. (Chimps are susceptible to infection but do not get AIDS; in any case, there is reluctance to use such an intelligent animal for this work and there is a world shortage of them.)

For these reasons, experts believe that a vaccine for routine use cannot be ready until the end of the century. This means that limitation of spread of the infection must depend on education.

It is not surprising that the AIDS epidemic has given rise to many claims of cure by the use of questionable medicines, that its sufferers have drawn heavily on the resources of alternative medicine and that in some cases cottage industries have arisen to produce spurious remedies. At the same time, the esoteric folklore that re-inforces the comradeship of infection labels as 'bad news' the use of chemotherapy and radiotherapy.

More reputable substances, many already known to be active against other viruses, have been tested *against the HIV itself* with little useful result. Only one drug has been found so far to be of real, if limited, value. This drug is Zidovudine (Retrovir, commonly known as AZT). In one test about 6 per cent of AIDS patients taking AZT had died after 9 months while about 40 per cent of patients not taking the drug had died. There many three points about the drug worth considering:

1. It is very expensive, costing about £7,000 per year per patient at today's prices.
2. It may prove toxic for some patients, damaging the red cell formation and causing severe muscle pains. Some doctors have reported having to take as many as 40 per cent of their patients off the drug because of this toxicity. However, perseverance and good management, including periodic blood transfusions, can make the treatment bearable.
3. Although it prolongs the patient's life in most cases, there is no evidence that the drug ever cures AIDS.

(AZT) overall tends to improve the quality of the patient's life and has some control over some of the more painful aspects of AIDS. It should be given in all cases when early symptoms occur (before the full AIDS picture emerges) and continued until the patient has no further expectation of a reasonable existence. At present a survey is commencing to evaluate the use of AZT in people early in HIV infection before any symptoms have appeared.

One of the difficulties in designing a drug for AIDS treatment is that the virus lives within the white cells responsible for maintaining immunity; any drug that destroyed the virus might well kill the white cells containing it and hence induce an artificial condition which is like AIDS.

Many of the opportunist organisms that cause infection in AIDS patients are amenable to treatment using antibiotics and similar substances and their skilful use can improve the quality of life in many cases.

Avoiding AIDS

AIDS is the best practical reason for monogamy. At present it is in the sphere of homosexual practice that this is most important but, if the spread among heterosexual becomes more common in the West, the need for heterosexual monogamy will increase; the current risks of contracting AIDS following a one-off contact in the West are lower than the chances of winning a football pool prize (but, we are assured, some people do win them!). Ideally, a life partnership should ensure safety.

For those who find this limitation of sexual activity tedious there are still a few options open. They may decide to cut out more hazardous types of sex and opt for mutual masturbation and other non-penetrative activities. If such alternatives are not attractive, then a condom should be used during sexual activity, with an especially stout one in genito-anal sex.

Those who are HIV positive should cut down their sexual activities in order to avoid both infecting their friends and catching any further sexually acquired infections. Women who are HIV positive should not become pregnant for two reasons. First, pregnancy can accelerate the onset of full-blown AIDS in HIV-infected women. Second, about 50 per cent of babies born to HIV- positive women are themselves infected, tending to develop AIDS and dying early in life.

Intravenous drug abusers should not share syringes or needles and local authorities should provide clean materials without appearing to condone the drug habit; they can comfort themselves that by doing this they are protecting others (e.g. consorts and offspring of drug takers) from HIV infection.

During visits to the Third World sex should be avoided, while travellers should carry an anti-AIDS kit which has a syringe and needle in case of emergency.

Hospital workers should treat all patients and blood specimens with respect, remembering that many cases of HIV (and other) infections are not labelled.

How infection is NOT spread

It is only after several years of public education that most of the general public have perceived the irrationality of their fears that they might contract AIDS by casual social contacts with sufferers. A newspaper report of the cremation of an early victim of the disease described how the body was wrapped in three layers of stout plastic, how the dead man's friends were not allowed into the crematorium chapel (presumably in case one of them had the infection and might leave the virus in the chapel to infect subsequent mourners) and how the furnace was operated at the temperature of the interior of the sun (an achievement that the world's greatest pysicists might envy!).

Since those days the situation has changed, mainly because of the sensible education policies pursued by the former Department of Health and Social Security. In the USA education in this matter has been less efficient, possibly because of the assumption of highly moral attitudes in a climate of born-again and fundamental Christianity, where words like homosexual cannot be used in public and condom has become the 'C-word'!

AIDS *is* a frightening disease and it is not surprising that those with little technical knowledge about it have taken extreme steps to prevent the infection in themselves and theirs, such as keeping their children away from a school where an HIV-positive haemophilic child was known to attend. It is very important to educate people, not only how to avoid HIV infection but also how not to disrupt their and other people's lives for fear of catching the disease.

HIV is not contracted by normal social contact, by shaking hands or by sharing crockery or from toilet seats or communion cups; it is not contracted by being coughed upon by infected persons or even by contact with their blood if the skin surface is intact. In the laboratory the handling of HIV-positive blood is less hazardous than handling blood contaminated by the hepatitis-B virus and gross carelessness is needed to contract infection from laboratory specimens.

The chances of contracting the disease from blood transfusion in or following the use of blood products are very small in the West now that testing of blood is carried out routinely and Factor 8 is heat treated; there should be few, if any, further cases of infection contracted in these ways.

Hepatitis B

The word 'hepatitis' denotes an infection of the liver. Several organisms can cause such an infection but the commonest two are the viruses that cause hepatitis A and hepatitis B.

Hepatitis and jaundice

The liver is the biggest organ in the body and it has a large number of functions so that liver failure leads rapidly to death. One function is to deal with superannuated red blood cells. These contain the red pigment haemoglobin which is altered in the liver to a yellowy-brown substance called 'bile pigment'. The bile pigment is produced in cells throughout the liver and it then passes along through tubes that become larger and larger, eventually reaching the gall bladder where it is stored and from which it eventually passes into the intestines through the bile duct. It is bile pigment that gives the normal stool its usual brown colour. (See Figure 7.7.)

If the bile pigment cannot reach the bowel it must go somewhere else and, in fact, it passes into the bloodstream and is carried all over the

Figure 7.7 Bile formation in the healthy liver

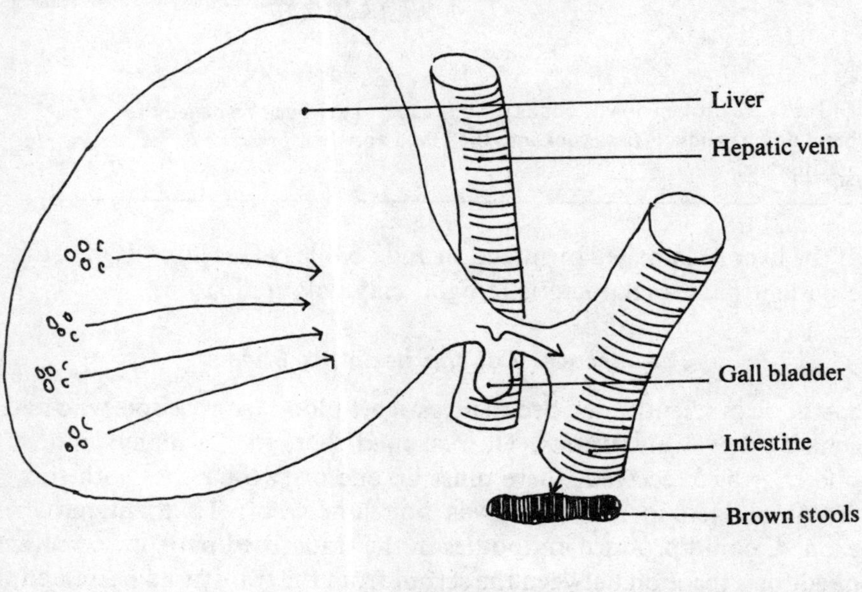

Old red cells are broken down and the breakdown products pass along the bile channels in the liver to the gall bladder and thence to the intestine via the bile duct.

body. Because it is yellow in colour, the skin and the whites of the eye also become yellow—this is the condition known as 'jaundice'. It is important to remember that, although jaundice is usually caused by liver damage, hepatitis frequently occurs without causing jaundice. (See Figure 7.8.)

Figure 7.8 Jaundice following liver damage

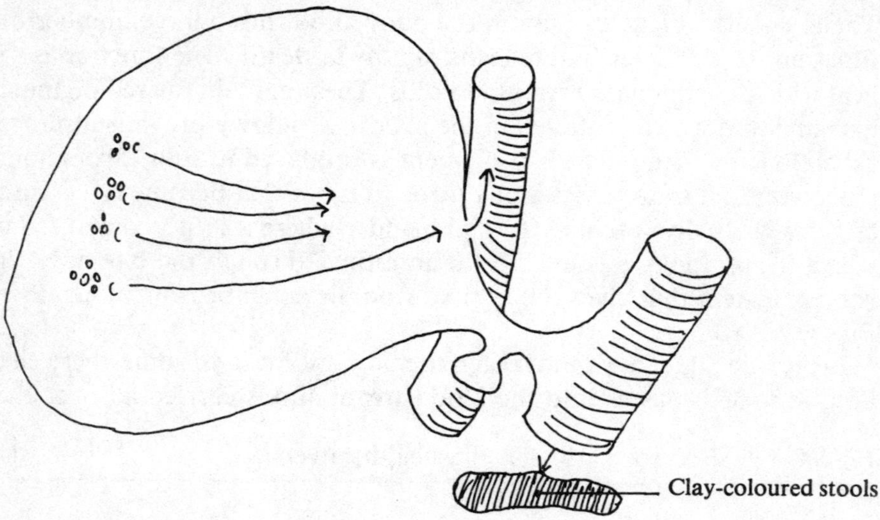

Old cells are broken down, but as the bile canals have been damaged the breakdown products pass back into the blood and their presence in the skin is seen as jaundice.

If the liver is damaged by infection and no bile passes into the intestine the patient passes characteristic light 'clay-coloured stools'.

The discovery of the hepatitis B virus

An American scientist decided to investigate blood from people who had received many transfusions. He reasoned that, in the many pints of blood they had received, there must be one or two batches with some unusual antigen in it but he was not sure what. That antigen, he reasoned, could produce antibodies in the transfused patient and so he looked for a reaction between the serum from the transfused person and various specimens of 'normal' blood.

He obtained one significant result: a reaction between his patient's blood and that from an Australian aborigine. Thus the substance in the Australian's blood was called Australia antigen and for many years the virus of hepatitis B was known as Australia antigen. It was soon found that the blood of other patients, particularly those suffering or recovering from hepatitis, reacted with the transfused patient's blood.

Figure 7.9 Hepatitis B

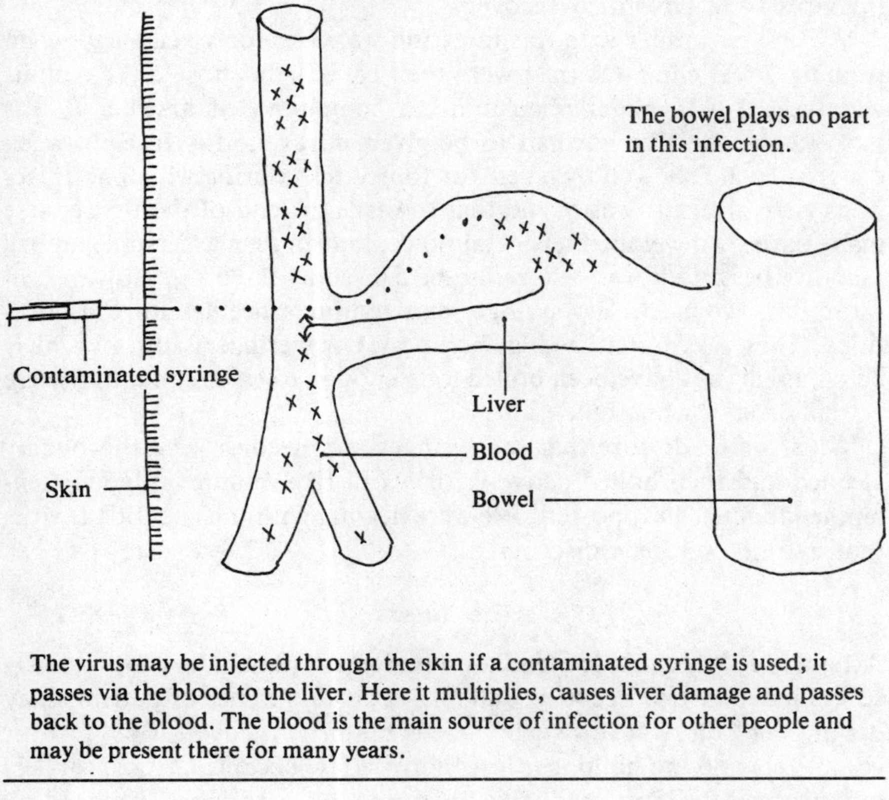

The virus may be injected through the skin if a contaminated syringe is used; it passes via the blood to the liver. Here it multiplies, causes liver damage and passes back to the blood. The blood is the main source of infection for other people and may be present there for many years.

Even before the Second World War it was suspected that there were two different kinds of virus hepatitis. Although clinically they were very similar, one type was rather more severe than the other and had a very long incubation period, up to three months. After the discovery of Australia antigen it was found that blood from patients with this sort of hepatitis gave a reaction like the patient with Australia antigen but patients with the other kind of hepatitis did not. Thus the two infections were called hepatitis A and hepatitis B to distinguish between them.

Mode of infection

It was eventually found that the virus of hepatitis B usually reached the blood either through homosexual activity or through the introduction of blood itself into the patient, perhaps by means of contaminated needles or through blood transfusion. (See Figure 7.9.) A disturbing thing about this disease was that, once infected, some patients could remain carriers for many years, although the majority of patients lost the virus soon after their recovery.

My first encounter with this infection was over forty years ago when running a VD clinic (as they were then called). In those days syphilis was treated with neoarsphenamine, a compound of arsenic. It was moderately effective but had to be given intravenously in eight-week courses, each followed by a rest for four weeks during which no injections were given. It was found that towards the end of the first course many patients developed severe jaundice, known then as 'arsphenamine' jaundice because it was believed to be caused by the drug. However, in those days we used glass syringes and re-usable needles for the injections. These were 'sterilized' in boiling-water sterilizers and, in a busy clinic, might not have been boiled long enough to ensure that they were actually sterile when taken out.

When we made sure that the syringes and needles *were* thoroughly cleaned and then boiled actively for a full five minutes, the arsphenamine jaundice disappeared! We were dealing with the hepatitis B virus that had not yet been discovered!

The illness

After a long but variable incubation period the patient develops a fairly severe jaundice and becomes quite ill. A small number of patients may die of liver failure at this stage but the majority recover. Most recover completely and are no longer infectious; a few become chronic carriers and in some the liver gradually becomes more and more damaged by the chronic infection, leading to death.

Cases and carriers

About 1,600 new cases and 100 new carriers are found in Britain each year and the carrier rate in the population is about 0.1 per cent. However, in some parts of the world the carrier rate may reach 25 per cent and the disease is a really serious matter. In Africa, for instance, there are millions of carriers. In that continent the incidence of cancer of the liver is very high indeed and it is the result of infection in childhood or at birth by the hepatitis B virus. It is here where mass vaccination would save tens of thousands of lives each year.

Avoiding hepatitis B

For most people there is no real danger of getting the infection. Like AIDS it seems to be mainly a disease of homosexuals and intravenous drug abusers; a particular danger is through syringe sharing by drug addicts. Those who deal with such patients, especially surgeons and dentists, and women married to chronic carriers may be at risk and there is something to be said for the vaccination of these groups. A safe vaccine is available and is made available to laboratory staff dealing with specimens from patients with the infection. The vaccine is made from the serum of patients with a heavy infection and hence carrying a lot of virus in the blood. This virus is killed by several different chemicals but is able still to stimulate the formation of antibodies.

In people with one-off risks, such as nurses who have pricked their fingers with a needle previously used on a hepatitis B patient, an antiserum is available with its ready-made antibody.

An important group of patients consists of babies born to women suffering from or carrying the virus of hepatitis B at delivery. These babies should be given the antiserum as soon as possible and also vaccinated within a day or so of birth.

Tattooing, ear piercing and acupuncture must be carried out under strictly hygienic conditions if hepatitis B is not to be transmitted. Hepatitis is very like AIDS in the way it spreads and the sort of people likely to develop it. Like AIDS, it is also an important disease in Africa; compared with that continent, the disease is a mere nuisance in the West.

Hepatitis C

It has been known for a long time that there are viruses other than those causing hepatitis A and hepatitis B capable of causing liver damage, especially following blood transfusion. Up until recently such viruses have been known, somewhat noncommitally, as 'Non-A' and 'Non-B' viruses. A short time ago a well-defined hepatitis virus, capable of causing what is now called hepatitis C, was discovered. There are, at present, no routine methods of identifying this virus; the current methods are so complicated that they can be carried out only in a high-powered research laboratory but enough has already been learned to indicate that hepatitis C is a very important disease.

We saw how hepatitis B was frequently contracted through blood transfusion and, in the case of haemophiliacs, from Factor 8. In the USA there are still large numbers of cases of hepatitis following transfusion; most of these seem to be caused by the hepatitis C virus.

There are about 150,000 cases of post-transfusion hepatitis annually in the USA. Half of these cases (75,000) go on to develop chronic hepatitis (and remain infectious); of these about 20 per cent (15,000) develop cirrhosis of the liver, which is usually fatal. Thus hepatitis C is probably responsible for around 10,000 deaths each year in that country.

In Britain there is evidence that 0.5 per cent to 1 per cent of blood donors (i.e. ordinary people) have evidence of previous infection (but are not necessary infectious). Intravenous drug addicts show evidence of infection in proportions varying from 48 per cent to 92 per cent, while for haemophiliacs the figures are 53 per cent 89 per cent.

Interestingly, specimens of Factor 8 (produced before heat treatment was the rule) that have given rise to jaundice in recipients have been found to contain the hepatitis C virus.

There are no methods at present for screening units of blood or blood donors on a large scale although methods are sure to be found in the next year or so, especially if hepatitis C proves to be as important an infection as it seems at present.

Herpes infections

This seems to be a good opportunity to recall the activities of the herpes group of viruses. These viruses all look identical, having tiny tubes on the surface and being enclosed in a membrane. There are a great number of types, many causing infection in animals, but only a few which are important to humans. These viruses all have the ability to remain in the body long after the infection has passed and often they re-appear to cause symptoms much later. *It must be emphasized that genital herpes is the only sexually acquired disease caused by the group*. (See Figure 7.10.)

The most important types of virus to humans are:

1. *Chickenpox virus*. This virus causes the normally very mild disease of chickenpox. After the patient has recovered, the virus remains in the body in the cells of the sensory nerves. When the patient is under stress or suffering from another kind of infection, the virus may pass down

the nerve fibres to the skin and cause crops of painful blisters, usually in elderly patients (shingles).

2. *Epstein-Barr virus*. This virus causes glandular fever and is associated with Burkitt's lymphoma in African children. The virus remains in certain white blood cells so that most patients who have been infected in the past are sporadically infectious. There are no recurrent symptoms caused by this virus.

3. *Cytomegalovirus*. This virus causes a very mild infection and is not important unless infection occurs in pregnancy or in patients with reduced immunity such as those suffering from AIDS. Women who

Figure 7.10 Types of herpes virus harboured by nerve cells in different parts of the spinal cord

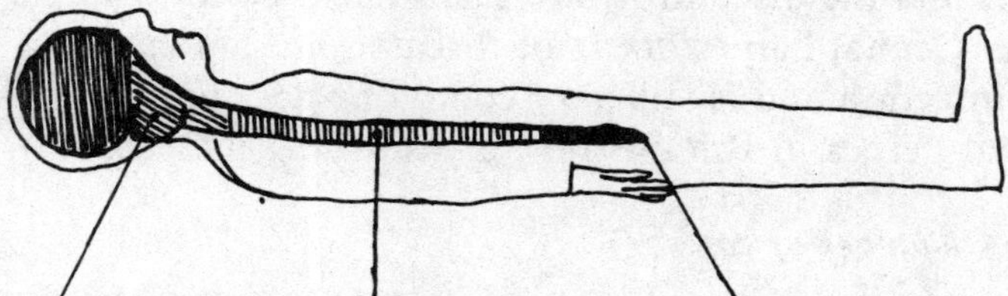

have been infected in the past may begin to excrete the virus again, especially during pregnancy, but this will not affect the baby as the mother's blood will contain antibody at this stage. The virus hibernates in white blood cells, certain large cells in the lining of the intestine and in other sites such as the salivary glands.

4. *Herpes simplex virus*. This virus infects almost everybody at some time. The commonest first infection is in the form of a severe mouth infection at the age of about four. This may take a week or so to heal and, when it does so, the virus takes refuge in the cells of the sensory nerves supplying the area originally infected and, at varying intervals, passing back along the nerve fibres to cause small blisters on the skin. The degree to which this occurs varies enormously: some people never have a recurrence; some have only one or two recurrences, especially in association with another, different infection ('cold sore'); while, in a few, the condition becomes a nightmare, recurring regularly every three months or even at shorter intervals. In some cases, especially in nurses and dentists, the first infection occurs later in life and on the hands as a result of contact with infected patients.

There are two types of herpes simplex. Type 1 was originally the cause of herpes lesions in the mouth, while type 2 was responsible for genital herpes; but our permissive society, by allowing a variety of sexual practices not even considered in the past, has blurred the edges of this distinction.

It is not clear whether infection with type 1 confers any immunity against infection with type 2 but it is said that the chances of catching genital herpes from an infected partner is about 80 per cent. In this infection the virus conceals itself in the cells of the nerve fibres supplying the sexual organs and, like the type 1 virus, passes down the nerve fibres to cause blisters around the original site of infection. Again, as with the superior form of herpes infection, many cases of first infections heal and never recur; but in some cases recurrence often happens and the frequency and the discomfort are such that they constitute a threat to marriage. Genital herpes does not threaten life but can be a most distressing infection and is still very commonplace. For example, figures for genital herpes in Britain show a disturbing increase:

Year	*Number of cases*
1979	9,576
1980	10,700
1982	14,042
1984	19,869

It should be pointed out that these are notified cases only; the true figures must be much greater.

We have already considered the importance of genital herpes in a mother near the time of delivery—the infection can be fatal to a new born baby. There is also a form of meningitis caused by this virus that occurs both in children and adults. The condition has a mortality rate of about 50 per cent and about half the survivors will have mental problems for life; fortunately this infection is not common.

Another important form of herpes infection occurs in children suffering from eczema. In such children the eczematic skin has little immunity; in the days when smallpox vaccination was carried out, instead of remaining localized, the 'take' would spread over all the eczematic skin, causing a superinfection that was often fatal. A similar condition, but caused by the herpes virus, can occur in a child with eczema if he contracts a herpes infection.

There are two other viruses which should be mentioned:

1. *Monkey B virus.* In monkeys this causes as mild an infection as

does herpes simpex in man. However the B virus occasionally affects humans, usually after monkey bites. In a recent incident four monkey handlers developed the infection and two died. Thus it is recommended that all who handle monkeys should wear protective clothing, including gloves, face mask and visor, and should shower after handling the animals. After a bite the wound should be washed thoroughly and allowed to bleed and a course of antiviral drugs should be given.
2. *Herpes virus 6.* This virus has been discovered during recent years and it seems to be the cause of a minor childhood infection, erythema subitum; in patients with deficient immunity it can cause an illness which is like glandular fever. It seems to be a well-adjusted parasite, infecting most people during their lifetime with little deleterious effect.

Avoiding herpes infection

There is no way of avoiding the primary mouth infection and it may be preferable not to try, because this infection provides a good measure of immunity to the infection in later life. If the condition becomes distressingly recurrent, it is often useful to use Acyclovir cream. This may be kept by the patient and applied at the very onset of the recurrence and will often abort the full-scale condition. The same is true of genital herpes, while the use of a condom during intercourse with a new partner is advisable.

Chlamydia

Chlamydia are tiny organisms resembling bacteria. The best known is the one that causes psittacosis (parrot disease), discussed in chapter 8.

Non-gonococcal urethritis

This is caused by strains of chlamydia differing from that causing psittacosis. After antibiotics became used widely for treatment gonorrhoea presented little problem; however, there remained an increasing number of men with a discharge from the urethra that did not contain recognizable bacteria and it was eventually found that this condition was caused by one of the chlamydia, the type discussed in Chapter 4. Occasionally a man may become infected with gonorrhoea and chlamydia at the same time. If the gonorrhoea is treated he will still have a discharge, but without gonococci. This condition is sometimes called post-gonococcal urethritis.

When symptoms do occur they consist of a painful urethral discharge in the man and a cervical discharge in the woman. The organism may also pass up the urinary tract; in the man the prostate and the epididymis (the sperm reservoir) may become infected. In women the organism infects the cervix, causing eye infections in babies as they are born. Because the uterus sheds its lining every month, this does not become infected but the organism can 'jump the gap' up to the Fallopian tubes. Here it can cause severe inflammation, resulting in pain and illness, and may also be responsible for some cases of sterility by causing blockage of these tubes. Surveys have shown that about 80 per cent of women in Britain have antibodies but two thirds of those infected have no symptoms.

There are several parallels between chlamydial infection and gonorrhoea:

1. In both cases men suffer urethritis and a discharge and the organisms may pass backwards to infect the prostate and epididymis.
2. In women the cervix and urethra is infected in both cases and both organisms can pass upwards to infect the Fallopian tubes causing sterility and chronic ill health 'pelvic sepsis'.
3. In both cases babies can contract eye infections during birth.

Avoidance and treatment of chlamydial infection

The recommended avoidance of promiscuity goes a long way towards keeping clear of infection and the use of a sheath with doubtful partners is recommended.

Although the sexually acquired infection is self-healing, the process can be speeded up by using the antibiotic tetracycline or one of its relatives.

EIGHT

Respiratory Infections

We now have to consider a little simple physiology. As we live and move we need energy for those purposes and this energy comes from burning glucose within our bodies. Nature might have used other sources of energy, such as radioactivity, but most living things on this planet depend upon energy released when oxygen is added to the sugar molecule. This may be called 'oxidation' or simply 'burning'. When we set fire to a lump of sugar we obtain energy at the cost of smoke, flame and a temperature high enough to damage human tissue. To avoid such a catastrophe living things have learned how to 'burn' in very small steps so that little or no heat is produced; but the energy from the glucose is made available in special energy-storing molecules which will release it when needed.

Whatever the form of burning used, both sugar and oxygen are needed at the site of oxidation. The sugar is absorbed from the intestine and reaches the blood which carries it, in solution, all over the body.

The problem of getting the oxygen to the right places (muscles, for instance) is more difficult; insects solve the problem by simply letting the oxygen dissolve in their body fluids; this is not a very efficient method because oxygen can diffuse only a little way in fluids and this is one reason why insects are comparatively small.

Higher animals have solved the problem by carrying the oxygen on haemoglobin or a similar substance. Haemoglobin is the red pigment in the red cells of the blood and it is able to form a *loose* combination with oxygen – not a *firm* chemical combination as in oxidation. When such combinations occur there is a tendency for oxygen to combine with the haemoglobin under conditions of high oxygen concentration and to part with it when the oxygen concentration is low. This is an ideal mechanism because in the lungs, where the oxygen tension is high as a result of the air inhaled, haemoglobin collects oxygen and carries it along in the blood until it reaches the muscles where the oxygen tension is low; here the haemoglobin gives up its oxygen and then returns to the lungs for more. During the whole of our lives our hearts pump the blood, first to the lungs and then to the body, to keep this oxygen cycle functioning. (See Figure 8.1.)

Figure 8.1 The oxygen cycle

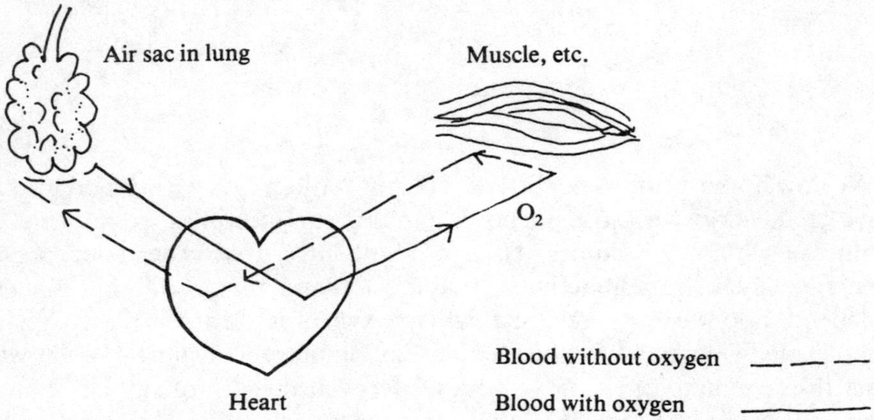

Blood collects oxygen from the lungs and is passed back to the heart. From here it is sent to the muscles and other organs; the oxygen they need is given up to them and the blood passes back again to the heart and thence to the lungs to collect more oxygen.

There are several penalties that man (and more especially, woman) has to pay for the privilege of walking in an erect position. One of these is a tendency to painful backs, another is the need for most women to wear bras and a third is the painful feet and distorted toes of women who wear high heels. Yet another is the tendency for our lungs to dangle down inside us, so that any fluid that they contain runs to the bottom of them rather than downwards and forwards as in a lower mammal. This has a bearing on chest infections, because one of the results of infection and inflammation is the outpouring of fluid. If the air-chambers of the lung, where the air and blood come into close contact and where the haemoglobin should pick up its oxygen, are full of fluid instead of air, then no oxygen can be collected. This results in a shortage of oxygen throughout the body that will cause illness and may result in death. (See Figure 8.2.)

We have seen how the cilia, combined with the mucus secreted by glands in the air passages, help to clear the lungs of unwelcome invaders. When the air passages become infected, one possible effect is damage to the cilia so that mucus is not 'flicked' upwards. (See Figure 8.3.) Another effect is damage to the muscle walls of the air passages so that they sag; 'bags' form in which all sorts of organisms can grow, making an internal and smelly sort of 'garden' – this condition is known as 'bronchiectasis'. (See Figure 8.4.) Such conditions may be caused by whooping cough, measles or tuberculosis.

Figure 8.2 The lungs in humans and animals

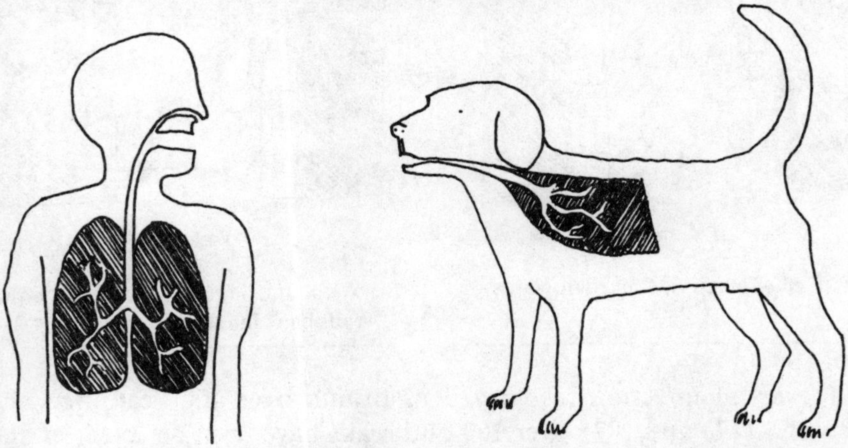

Influenza: the last plague

In 1567 an English physician wrote:

> It began with a roughness of the jaws (sore throat), small cough and then a strong fever, with a pain of the head, back and legs; some felt as though they were corded over the heart and had a weight on the stomach; all which continued to the third day at the farthest; then the fever went off with a sweat or bleeding at the nose. In some few it turned to a pleurisy or a fatal peripneumony.

This is an account of influenza which would serve today. The disease was called influenza because it was believed caused by the 'influence' of the sun, moon and planets, although this astrological explanation has yet to be confirmed.

Figure 8.3 Loss of cilia from bronchial lining

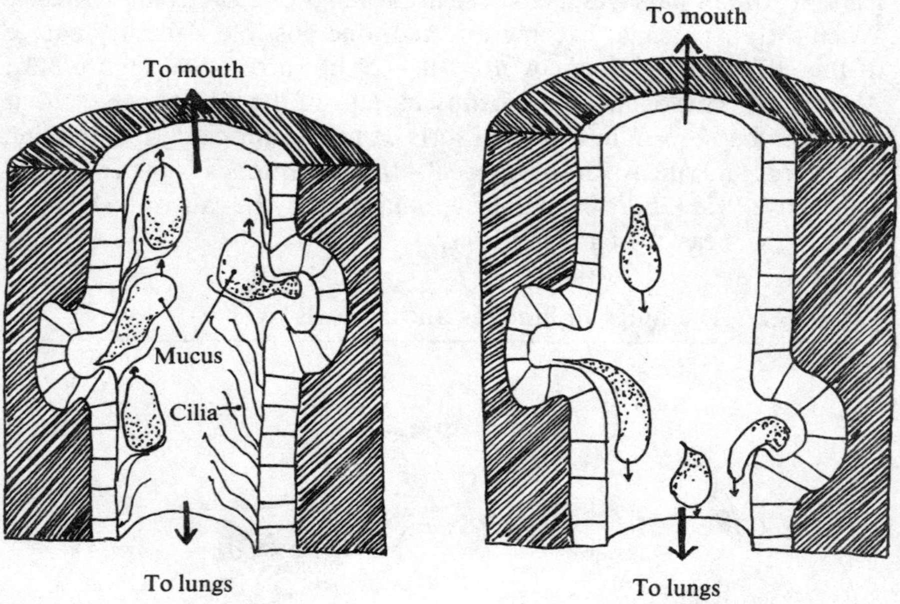

With cilia, mucus is flicked upwards.

Without cilia, mucus (and organisms) falls back into the lungs.

It was an infection recognized in Britain over 400 years ago and between 1173 and 1875 over 300 outbreaks have been detected, at and average interval of 2.4 years. Some of these outbreaks have been disastrous; for instance, in 1426–7 an outbreak affected what is now Spain, France, the Netherlands and Britain and in eastern England about 5 per cent of the population died.

At the same time as influenza, a similar but distinct infection known as the Sweating Sickness or the Picardy Sweat affected western Europe. This was a disease of sudden onset, often killing within six hours. In September and October 1485 two mayors of London and four aldermen died of it and it seemed to attack the young and rich rather than the old and poor. We shall never now know its cause – it might have been a severe form of influenza but most experts believe otherwise.

The word 'influenza' or 'flu' is often used loosely, especially by doctors who realize that they do not and probably never will know the exact cause of a patient's respiratory infection. There are a vast number of viruses (and bacteria) capable of causing mild respiratory illness and it is rarely cost effective to investigate such illnesses. However, the term 'flu' is not very appropriate for mild respiratory infections, partly because there is little 'catarrh' in the early stage of true influenza and also because it is a very unpleasant disease.

The illness

Onset is sudden and patients can often give its exact time. They feel very ill and develop a temperature with shivering and a dry cough with pain behind the breastbone. After a while the cough becomes 'productive' and the patient may even feel that he is coughing up part of his lung. In most cases after three days the temperature settles and most patients begin to feel better, although some may remain ill for up to ten days.

Figure 8.4 Bronchiectasis

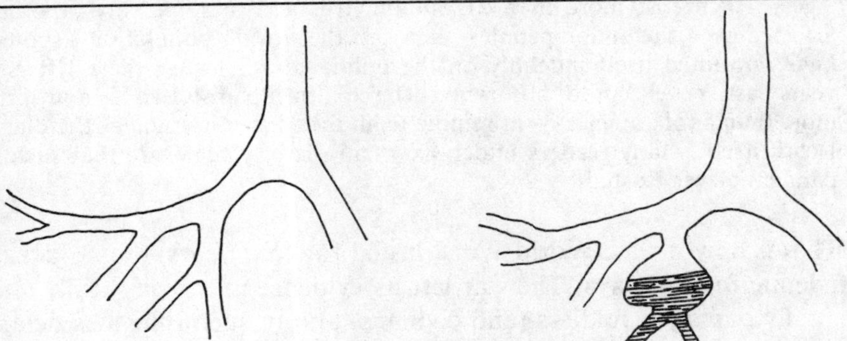

Normal bronchi

Abnormal bronchi
The bronchi have been widened and harbour infected fluid that can spread to other parts of the lung.

Outbreaks of influenza

We have seen that, in the past at least, most western countries have outbreaks of influenza every few years; these are usually quite small but, nevertheless, kill a number of elderly people and also some patients with chronic diseases such as diabetes or kidney trouble. However, at irregular intervals a pandemic takes place that sweeps over the world; the mortality rate is not usually high but, because of the sheer number of cases, the number of deaths is enormous. Such pandemics occurred in 1836, 1847, 1889 and, of course, in 1918.

The pandemic of 1918

Pandemics have occurred since, but none having the terrible effect of that of 1918. It has to be remembered that World War I was still in progress when the first wave of infection took place in September 1918. The pandemic went on until December 1918, with three separate waves. In October alone 400,000 Americans died from the infection. The whole outbreak killed at least 21,000,000 people throughout the world and the total sick were about 500,000,000 – about half the world population. About three times as many died from influenza as were killed in the war. Writing in 1974, one writer says:

> Perhaps the most puzzling factor about the Spanish Lady was her impermanence. On the face of it, the most appalling epidemic since the Middle Ages, which cost more than 21 million lives and in some way or other affected over one billion people – then half the world's population – should have imprinted itself indelibly on the public consciousness these fifty-six years past. Yet except to those who suffered it the Spanish Lady is now little more than a folk memory – as remote from the conscious mind as the Black Death itself. Many readers under sixty can scarcely be aware that such a pandemic ever existed.

That is how it was: World War I lasted for four years, the influenza pandemic for 120 days. The war left its evidence in the physically and mentally damaged soldiers (and civilians) and in such things as debts, reparations and boundary changes, while those attacked by the Spanish Lady had short illnesses from which they either died or recovered. For this reason a disaster – by the side of which our potential AIDS epidemic seems little more than a mild nuisance – has practically disappeared from the world's memory and its history books.

Preventing influenza

Influenza is caused by a virus which resembles that causing mumps. It has some superficial resemblance to the AIDS virus in that it can alter its surface. As we have seen, the surfaces of organisms carry certain substances (antigens) that stimulate the formation of antibodies that make the subject immune to further infection by that organism. Thus, when a patient has already had hepatitis A he does not catch it again. Influenza type A (the type responsible for pandemics and other large outbreaks) has the ability to change the substances in its surface, sometimes slightly (*antigenic drift*) and sometimes greatly (*antigenic shift*). (See Figure 8.5.)

Figure 8.5 Influenza A – antigenic shift

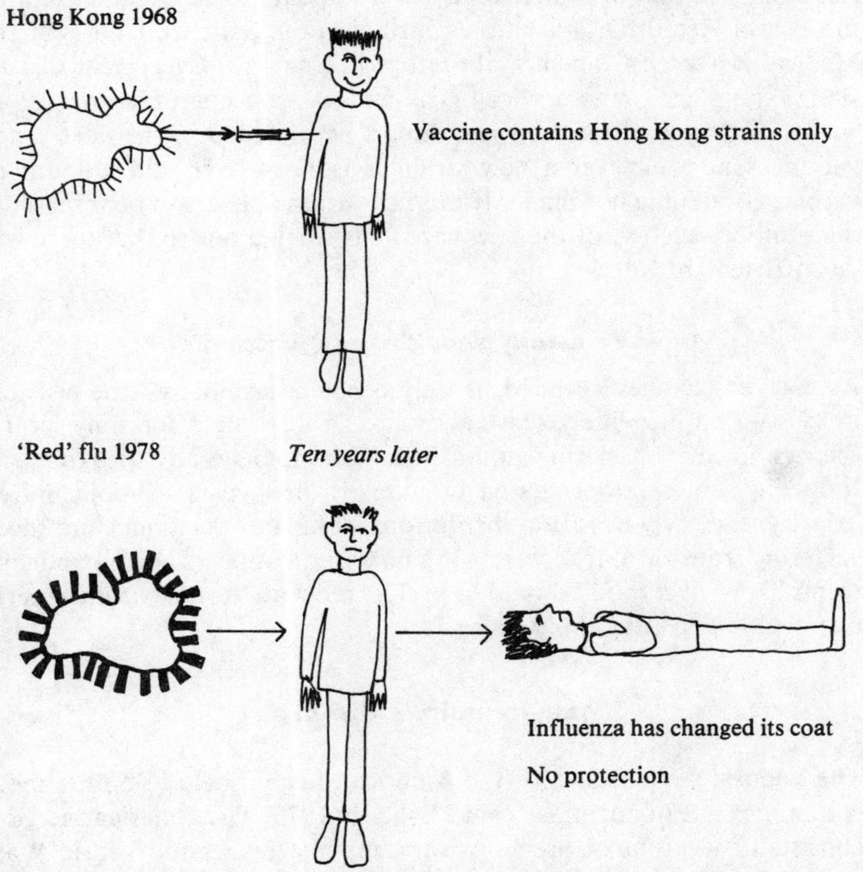

Thus we can experience a pandemic of a new sort of flu A which spreads all over the world. All who become infected by this strain become immune to it (providing that they survive) so for the next few years only a few (i.e. those that missed the first wave) become infected each year. Then, several years after the first wave a flu virus may appear with a slightly different surface; those people with antibody to the old flu A find that it is of no protective value and they may become infected with the new variety, which gradually takes the place of the old strain until yet another different strain occurs in a few years time.

Because of the flu virus's ability to change its surface antigen, any vaccine given must, of course, be made from the current (new) strains.

For this reason, there are all over the world laboratories constantly examining strains of flu isolated from patients. The headquarters of the World Health Organization's Influenza Surveillance Unit is at the Medical Research Council's laboratory in England. Every year discussions take place between virologists and vaccine manufacturers as to which strains of influenza virus should be included in the next year's vaccines and whenever a new strain is isolated a certain amount of vaccine containing it is made. If this new strain appears to be spreading, then full production of the new vaccine is carried out so that there will be sufficient for all.

How frequently should we be vaccinated?

As marked changes in the virus only occur occasionally—the last was in 1978—and it is likely that vaccination will protect for some years, there is no call for routine annual vaccination. Generally speaking, the following should be vaccinated about every three years: school children over eight, elderly people in institutions, some key personnel and those suffering from chronic diseases. If a new strain appears and a pandemic seems likely, everybody should be vaccinated with the new strain as early as possible and preferably twice.

Legionnaire's disease

The Pennsylvania branch of the American Legion held its 58th annual conference in Philadelphia from 21–4 July 1976. The American Legion consists of veterans of previous wars, mainly the Second World War, and their spouses; the institution resembles the British Legion but is rather more up-market. The conference included meetings for all delegates, a parade, a testimonial dinner, a dance, committee meetings, regional sub-meetings and a breakfast and there were also activities in the large hotel lobby and several meeting rooms. As the majority present were ex-soldiers at a re-union, it is likely that the flow of whisky and beer was not restricted.

Soon after the meeting 182 of those who had attended the reunion became ill with signs of pneumonia and, by the time that the final figures were obtained, twenty-nine had died. These figures were not easy to obtain because most of those who became ill did so after returning to their homes which were scattered around the state.

This seemed to be another new disease and, typically, the US health authorities left no stone unturned in efforts to identify the cause of the outbreak. There were many suggestions but the most likely cause seemed to be a virus. However, after several months of exhaustive study, it was found that, using a staining method so old that it was no longer in the textbooks, the lungs of guinea-pigs who had been injected with material from fatal cases of the disease were full of small bacteria. It was later found that the organism could be *grown* by using the most nutritious medium available.

Once it was possible to grow the organism it was possible to look for antibody toward it in patients and others. All those who had the clinical infection had such antibody but also many of the people employed in the hotel concerned also had antibody. Another approach was the examination of blood serum taken from patients in earlier unexplained outbreaks of respiratory infection for antibody to this organism, now known as Legionella.

Such antibody was present in patients from several outbreaks, including the outbreak of so-called Pontiac fever, which was associated with a public building in the town of Pontiac in Michigan. This illness had resembled a very mild attack of influenza and there had been no deaths.

Going even further back, an organism had been isolated in 1947 – almost thirty years earlier – from a man with mild pneumonia, and this was now identified as resembling that causing the Philadelphia outbreak.

Because of the great publicity surrounding the latter, the condition was labelled Legionnaire's disease and the organism responsible was called *Legionella pneumophilia* ('pneumophilia' means 'fond of lungs'). It is now known that there are many related organisms and that they can grow quite freely in most collections of static water if the temperature is right. For instance, the organism was isolated in a creek near a student's union complex where cases had occurred. It has also been found in cooling towers and faulty air conditioning systems and may also occur in parts of shower heads and other plumbing devices. The organism has frequently been found in domestic water supplies in hospitals and hotels. In hotels, where only a few or odd sporadic cases occur, it is likely that the showers may disseminate the infection, while in hospitals it has been quite often the cooling towers at fault.

One of the most recent outbreaks was at Stafford in England in 1985, when 101 people became ill and twenty-eight died. This was the next largest outbreak to the original one in the USA. In January the hospital engineers heard the Legionella had been found in the pond of one of the hospital's four cooling towers; some efforts were made to purify the water but these were not up to the standard required by the Department of Health and Social Security. In April the outbreak occurred but by the nineteenth of that month the dissemination of the organism had stopped, i.e. before the outbreak had been recognized.

The illness

Infection by Legionella may cause any degree of illness between mild 'flu' and death. A common sequence of events is:

1. Mild 'flu' with temperature, headache and muscle pains.
2. A progressive dry cough.
3. Some diarrhoea in 60 per cent of cases.
4. Some degree of mental upset with hallucinations or dizziness.

The disease responds to antibiotics, particularly erythromycin, and this is given to all cases of pneumonia of doubtful cause, because laboratory confirmation of the diagnosis may take a week or so and nothing is lost should the diagnosis not be Legionnaire's disease. Cure is preferable to accurate diagnosis.

Tuberculosis

Tuberculosis is a disease of great antiquity caused almost exclusively by one of the two main tubercle bacilli—the human or the bovine variety—both of which infect humans. Tubercle bacilli are small and slow growing but they stain very distinctly and, if seen in smears of sputum, are sufficiently characteristic as to warrant immediate treatment with the appropriate antibiotics before the diagnosis is finally clinched by actually growing the organism.

Although we usually think of tuberculosis of the *lungs* when we use the word 'tuberculosis' by itself, these bacilli can, in fact, affect almost any part of the body. In the past we have seen tuberculosis of the lungs, the lymph glands, the bones (especially the spine), the kidneys, the bowel, tuberculous meningitis and a widespread version referred to as military tuberculosis.

Pulmonary tuberculosis

Pulmonary tuberculosis is contracted by inhaling live tubercle bacilli, nearly always from a patient who is coughing them up. On the whole sufferers from pulmonary tuberculosis are not highly infectious but at some stages may be so—so-called 'open' cases—and these are responsible for the spread of pulmonary tuberculosis throughout the community.

1. *Primary tuberculosis.* This refers to the first infection, when the inhaled tubercle bacilli multiply in the cells of the lungs, forming a small abscess. In most people this heals, becomes impregnated with calcium and can be seen on X-rays as a dark spot at the top of one of the lungs. In a few cases the illness may run a rapid and fatal course.
2. *Reinfection.* After the primary infection most people are immune to further infection but a small number later develop a re-infection which tends to spread through the lung. (The disease may progress particularly rapidly in people with reduced immunity, especially AIDS patients.)

The efficient use of antibiotics (beginning with streptomycin) has practically abolished all but the occasional undiscovered case of *chronic* tuberculosis, which thirty or more years ago was the most common form of the infection. It consisted of a slow, grinding war between the disease and the patient's immune mechanism.

The small abscess first formed would enlarge and then leak into one of the air passages. This would enable the patient to cough up the contents of the abscess (and probably to infect a few more people in the process) and leave behind a cavity—a spherical hole in which all sorts of other organisms could multiply. The cavity would be walled off with fibrous tissue and the whole complex would remove a fair proportion of lung from its proper function of active respiration.

The disease might then either remain static for a time or progress to produce more and larger cavities, while all the time the patient would suffer from increasing weakness and 'night sweats'. If the abscess ate into small blood vessels the sputum would be bloodstained and, when it damaged a large artery, severe and perhaps fatal haemorrhage might follow. (See Figure 8.6.) Sometimes the abscess 'leaked' into blood vessels and tubercle bacilli were carried all over the body. These would produce small abscesses throughout the body, visible on x-rays as 'miliary tuberculosis', and sometimes localized abscesses, perhaps in the brain.

Patients died quite slowly, their illnesses frequently lasting for years and their deaths spreading over two or more days. Because of the gradual and remorseless course of the illness in its later stages, tuberculosis was a favourite disease with novelists and opera librettists.

As we shall see, the picture of tuberculous infection has changed radically and it may soon loom as small in the public eye as does the 1918 influenza outbreak today. In 1838 when figures were first collected there were about 30,000 deaths per year, making up about 17 per cent of all deaths. In 1954 the deaths were only about 4 per cent of those in 1838 and in 1979 they were down to about 0.5 per cent. Much of this improvement has been due to improvements in conditions of living – moving, as it were, out of the Third World. An additional impetus to the fall in mortality was the discovery of streptomycin and the development of other drugs which has made the fall after 1947 much steeper.

Figure 8.6 A tuberculous abscess 'eats into' an artery and causes severe haemorrhage

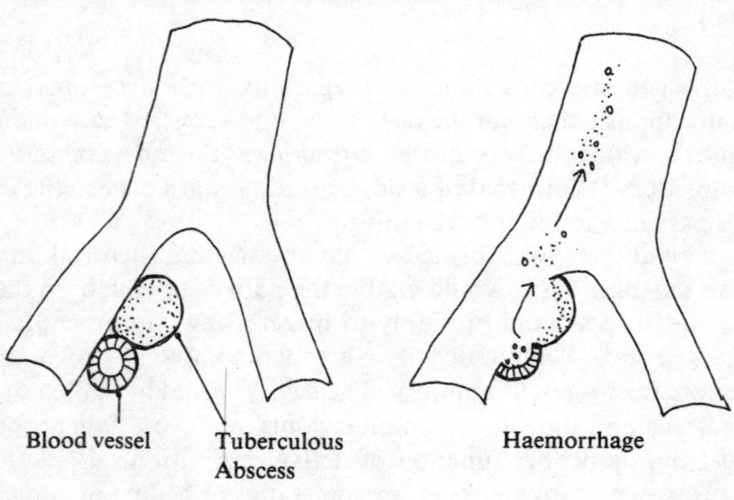

During the earlier years of this century certain doctors were appointed as Tuberculosis Officers by local authorities and their sole duty was to treat and investigate cases of tuberculosis. Before the advent of streptomycin, treatment consisted mainly of rest, fresh air, good food and methods of paralysing the affected lung in order to rest it if the infection was confined to one side only. There were also more bizarre forms of treatment; one County Tuberculosis Officer I knew used to prescribe *brass enemas* (fortunately the brass was in powder form!) and was positive that the infection came from the soil.

My abiding picture of the bad old days of tuberculosis is one of a row of hospital beds, each occupied by a gaunt emaciated wreck of what once was a woman. Around each, in the drizzly twilight of the northern town, their relatives sit, the men in their best serge suits, hopeless and feeling useless, wondering, perhaps, if it would be disrespectful to light a cigarette at this time. I must admit that, when I felt that I and the relatives had had enough (the patient by then having sunk into her final unconsciousness and not able to be consulted), I frequently prescribed, on my night rounds, a healthy dose of morphia so that the patient passed gently away before morning. It was then that I began to understand that a doctor's duty is not only to heal the sick but also to make the dying comfortable.

Bovine tuberculosis

Bovine tuberculosis is the strain of tubercle bacillus that infects cattle but humans are practically as susceptible as the animals. Cows suffering from this infection excrete the tubercle bacilli in their milk. When this is swallowed by humans the milk neutralizes the acid in the stomach and makes it easier for the tubercle bacilli to pass through to the intestine.

Robert Koch was a great German scientist who discovered the tubercle bacillus and who practically invented the science of bacteriology. However, he was sometimes over-dogmatic when speaking on subjects about which he was not completely informed. In 1901 he asserted with confidence that the bovine tubercle bacillus did not affect man. This was known at that time by most experts to be untrue but Koch was held in such high esteem that it was another twenty or thirty years before pasteurization of milk was introduced. (Until then the wise boiled their milk before use!) Thus, during that period, thousands of people developed intestinal, glandular and spinal tuberculosis and thousands died because of the inaccurate statements of an otherwise great man. Unfortunately, the tendency to regard as the gospel truth any statement by an eminent man on a subject with which he is not familiar is still a common human habit.

Tests for tuberculosis

These are the following tests for tuberculosis:

1. *Tuberculin tests.* It was shown quite early that if an extract of tubercle bacilli was injected into the skin of a patient, a raised red patch would appear if the patient had already been infected by the tubercle bacillus. Thus people who had already suffered their primary (first) infections and who were presumably immune would give a positive tuberculin test. Two variants of this test are the Mantoux and the Heaf tests (simply different ways of getting tuberculin into the skin).

In my generation almost all people had positive tests by the age of twenty-five but the percentages have now decreased, especially in the young.

A similar test is used in the maintenance of tuberculosis free cattle.

2. *Mass miniature x-rays.* Soon after the Second World war real efforts were made at last to stamp out tuberculosis in Britain. One of these was the introduction of Mass Miniature X-ray Units. These were vans that toured the whole country carrying small x-ray machines and they offered the public free chest x-rays. If the small chest x-ray looked suspicious the subject was sent to a chest clinic where he was examined by a chest physician and a full size x-ray taken. These units were very useful in the early days but, as the numbers of cases of tuberculosis in the public dwindled, the mass miniature x-ray units ceased to be cost-effective. To pick up one case of tuberculosis in 1,000 x-rays might be satisfactory but, when the proportion fell to one case in 10,000 examinations, the exercise ceased to be worthwhile.

Vaccination against tuberculosis

As soon as Koch had discovered the tubercle bacillus, the race was on to produce a vaccine but it quickly became clear that it would have to be a live vaccine—extracts of tubercle bacilli such as tuberculin did not produce immunity.

Two French workers, Albert Calmette and Camille Guérin, began in 1908 with a virulent strain of the organism isolated from a cow's udder. Painstakingly, they subcultured this strain every four to five weeks over many years. In 1914 the First World War began but they carried on with their work even though their town, Lille, was occupied by the Germans. In 1924, after sixteen years of work the organism they were now working with had become quite different from the one with which they had started and was stable—unlikely to change. This was the Bacillus Calmette–Guérin (BCG).

France at once embarked with great and patriotic enthusiasm on a programme for vaccinating children against tuberculosis with BCG but doctors in other countries were sceptical. To make matters worse, in 1930 in Lubeck in northern Germany, 249 ten-day-old babies were given oral BCG and sixty-seven died of acute tuberculosis; on investigation it was found that a virulent culture of tubercle bacilli had been stored in the same refrigerator as the BCG and used by mistake.

The value of BCG vaccination was not accurately measured until a British Medical Research Council trial was reported in 1956, showing that unvaccinated children were six times more likely to contract tuberculosis than vaccinated ones. Since then BCG has been used routinely in schoolchildren who have a negative skin test and are apparently susceptible to tuberculous infection.

As the incidence of tuberculosis falls even lower in Britain, the need for routine BCG vaccination becomes more questionable; however, it is certainly useful for skin test negative contacts of known cases and also for children of ethnic minorities, who seem more susceptible. In poorer countries BCG vaccine at birth is one of the most successful methods of controlling tuberculosis, not to mention the cheapest.

Tuberculosis may no longer be an infection of great significance in Britain but, worldwide, there are about 13 million cases of tuberculosis and about 3 million patients die annually.

Other respiratory infections

There are many other respiratory infections, caused mainly by bacteria or viruses, but most are relatively mild. Four conditions that may still be serious may be of interest:

Lobar pneumonia
Bronchopneumonia
Mycoplasma infection
Psittacosis

Lobar pneumonia

This disease is now rare in Britain but still occurs in the USA and may still occur in poorer countries. It is caused by a cousin of the streptococcus that causes tonsillitis, known as the *Streptococcus pneumoniae*. Before the days of penicillin lobar pneumonia would appear out of the blue, affecting and often killing young adults in the prime of life.

After chest pains, a cough and a high temperature the patient might lapse into a coma, remaining unconscious for a few days; he then either died or broke into a gentle perspiration and woke up practically recovered. Like tuberculosis, lobar pneumonia was a favourite disease for novelists – the heroine sitting by the hero's bedside until, after several days of restless coma, he awoke and asked: 'Where am I?' (Alternatively, if it was opportune to write him out, he did not wake up!) Now that antibiotics are immediately available for most patients, it has meant that the disease has practically disappeared in many countries.

Bronchopneumonia

When a patient suffering from a severe illness such as terminal cancer, a stroke or senility becomes so weak as to be unable to cough up the fluids that inevitably accumulate in his chest, many normally harmless organisms multiply in that fluid, causing further infection and the formation of more pus and fluid until the patient dies gently from lack of oxygen.

Although, when dealing with younger subjects with curable diseases, this type of pneumonia can often be treated with suitable antibiotics, in intractable cases – the very ill and the very old – a caring physician will rarely intervene, allowing the 'old people's friend' to supply the old people's need.

Mycoplasma infection

I sometimes wonder if this condition is so little known to the general public because of its outlandish name. It is, in fact, the commonest cause of mild pneumonia in Britain and about 40 per cent of school leavers have antibodies towards this organism, showing that they have been infected at some time. It causes a spectrum of symptoms extending from the unexpected to the unpleasant. It almost never causes death and recovery from the illness – if, indeed, the infection elicited symptoms – is usually rapid and may be speeded up with antibiotics.

The illness is caused by a small bacterium that has lost its cell wall; this renders it quite 'plastic', enabling it to squeeze through filters that will hold back respectable bacteria. For this reason it was thought to be a virus and given the noncommittal name 'Eaton's agent'; its present name is *Mycoplasma pneumoniae*.

Psittacosis

In 1928 I persuaded my parents to buy a parrot which we of course called Polly (we never discovered its sex). A little later we were upset to read of outbreaks of 'parrot disease' in people dealing with parrots imported from various parts of the world. This quite often caused a fatal pneumonia because, in those days, there were no antibiotics to effect cures. After that time the importation of parrots was spasmodically restricted.

It was eventually discovered that the disease was caused by a strain of chlamydia distinct from that causing the sexually acquired variety of infection. The infection still occurs from time to time but seems much milder than it used to be and it may be associated with budgerigars, pigeons and other birds. I have seen a case in an ardent budgerigar fancier who was so concerned about one of his sick birds that he gave it the kiss of life!

On another occasion a colleague was investigating a small outbreak of mild psittacosis in a celebrated British public school. There seemed to be no connection with parrots or budgerigars but tactful investigations revealed that some of the senior boys were in the habit of retiring to a nearby ruined church tower for a quiet smoke. The tower was also frequented by pigeons and it was shown that some of these carried the psittacosis virus.

It is obvious from the above that it is not now easy to acquire psittacosis, but steps to avoid possible infection include omitting to give the kiss of life to an ailing psittacine bird and also taking great care in choosing a suitable place for a quiet smoke!

Polly lived a long and rather blasphemous life, eventually becoming a victim to smoke from a kitchen fire about thirty years after her purchase!

The common cold

This disease is a nuisance and, although it affects the respiratory tract, it is not really a chest infection; however, this seems the best place to deal with it.

The 'cold' is so called because it was believed that the condition was brought about by exposure to unduly low temperatures. This is not entirely true because all colds are the result of infection of the membrane lining the nose; the inside of the nose is irritated and this causes sneezing. The purpose of a sneeze is to clear the nose of obstruction but, in most cases, any obstruction is caused by swelling of the lining membrane and the only effect of the sneeze is to spread the causative virus far and wide. Exposure to cold may play some part in that it might reduce the person's immunity at the time he came into contact with the virus.

The common cold is the commonest cause of absence from work and probably also the commonest excuse for this. In the USA it is the commonest cause of the patient visiting his doctor but in Britain I believe that this occurs mainly when a certificate is needed.

A large variety of viruses have been found to cause a cold-like illness.

Many of these viruses were also capable of causing other kinds of illness, such as diarrhoea, muscle pains, a rash and even mild meningitis. Later, an astute virologist realized that the nose projects a variable but definite distance in front of the face; he took temperatures of noses and found them to be several degrees lower than the temperature of the rest of the body. This encouraged him to incubate nasal secretions in tissue culture at lower temperatures than was usual and this procedure led to the isolation of a new group of viruses known either as 'coryzaviruses' (cold viruses) or 'rhinoviruses' (nose viruses). An embarrassing number of 'cold' viruses—well over one hundred—have now been discovered and, because such a large number of strains would need to be included, it is not possible to produce an effective vaccine.

The Common Cold Unit in Salisbury in England, alas no longer with us, functioned as a centre for the investigation of the ways that colds spread ever since the USA handed it over to the British Ministry of Health soon after the end of the Second World War. Much work has been carried out both there and in the USA and, although a lot has been learned, some of it seems almost contradictory.

In some instances it seemed that cold viruses might be spread from contaminated hands but this seems likely only in those with low levels of hygiene such as babies or toddlers. It has been shown by concealed video cameras that even the most fastidious people have a tendency to pick or rub their noses when not aware they are being observed. However, a perceptive critic suggested that this would be insufficient to spread the virus; to do so they would need to pick other people's noses, which they were not observed to do!

Such is the devotion to the progress of medical science that a number of miniature field trials have been carried out in the name of the epidemiology of the common cold. These are really 12-hour poker games with half the players suffering from deliberately induced streaming colds and the other half uninfected persons who are susceptible because they had no antibody to the virus causing the colds in their playmates. In some cases the uninfected players were fitted with wooden collars a metre wide to prevent close contact with the infected players. This precaution did not prevent infection: 56 per cent of the 'uncollared' group became infected and 67 per cent of the 'collared'. Many experiments have been carried out in huts in which the infected persons are segregated at one end, separated from the uninfected by wire netting; air flow was encouraged by the use of fans. In nearly every experiment infection was passed from the infected to the uninfected, suggesting 'droplet spread'.

In view of the almost certain fact that colds are spread by droplets, it is polite to segregate oneself during the 'streaming' phase and, despite what has been said, the use of tissues impregnated with a bactericidal substance seems to reduce the risk of spread of the infection. One can only treat the symptoms, not the underlying infection; while the nose is blocked it is wise to administer decongestant drops at regular intervals but to stop using them as soon as the passages become clear. Bed rest and aspirins (for adults), warm saline gargles for sore throats and codeine may be needed to suppress a painful cough.

It is said that a lady visited her doctor in January because she had a cold. The doctor suggested that she should take all her clothes off and stand at an open window. 'But, Doctor', she exclaimed, 'I might catch pneumonia!' 'Pneumonia', he replied, 'I can cure, but not a common cold!'

NINE

Bowel Infections

It was Tom Lehrer who said, many years ago, that life was like a sewer; what you get out of it depends on what you put into it. This is also true of the human bowel, with the added proviso that what you put into it may also affect the speed at which something comes out of it. One needs only to look around when one or two are gathered together to eat to be reminded how close we still are to earthworms, our main activity consisting of taking in energy-rich material at one end and rejecting the useless residue at the other end, more or less at a time of our own choosing. If in our intake of food and water there happens to be a sufficient number of capable organisms, the result is what we know as diarrhoea.

A definition of diarrhoea is 'bowel movements that are too frequent or too fluid' and both these factors allow of more effective transmission of the causative organisms to other people.

As well as diseases directly infecting the alimentary tract, other organisms or their products, taken by mouth, can affect more remote parts of the body; thus the hepatitis A virus can affect the liver and cause jaundice, the poliovirus may cause paralysis—as can also the toxin of *Clostridium botulinum*.

Organisms responsible

The important pathogens acquired by mouth are:

1. *Bacteria*.
The bacteria which cause actual infection of the lining of the bowel, multiplying in it and causing damage, include

Shigella (the family of dysentery organisms),

Salmonella (typhoid and food poisoning) and
Campylobacter.

The organisms which do not *infect* but multiply in the contaminated food and produce a toxin that causes illness include
Staphylococcus aureus,
Cl. welchii (Cl. perfringens),
Bacillus cereus and
Cl. botulinum.

2. *Protozoa*, which include
Giardia lamblia,
Entamoeba histolytica and
Cryptosporidium.

3. Viruses, which include
Norwalk virus,
Rotavirus and
Hepatitis A virus.

These are only some of the viruses that cause infection via the bowel; there are certainly many more. However, looking for viruses is a complicated and costly business and is carried out only in cases of large or important outbreaks of bowel infection. The ways in which bowel infections are spread was discussed in Chapter 2 and further information is given later in this chapter when discussing outbreaks.

Diarrhoea

We all know what diarrhoea is and it has been defined as the passage of too frequent or too fluid stools; it can be thought of as the attempt by the bowel to dilute and to expel any irritating substances that may be within it. Severe diarrhoea may occur in cholera, for instance, when the stool may be completely fluid, being mainly a solution of salts but containing many organisms; it may contain as many as 1,000,000,000 organisms per millilitre. Thus, severe diarrhoea can reduce both water and salt reserves of the body and this can be seen in the emaciation and sunken eyes of those with such diarrhoea. The water excreted must come from somewhere and does, indeed, come from the blood. Normal blood consists of 45 per cent cells and 55 per cent liquid (plasma); following severe diarrhoea these figures may be reversed. The increased amount of red cells makes the blood thicker and more liable to clot, causing thrombosis in the veins. (See Figure 9.1.)

The loss of salts in the fluid stools has a severe effect and leads to further dehydration; thus, in order to treat diarrhoea it is necessary not only to give water but also salts. In a developed country a patient with severe diarrhoea would be in hospital receiving an intravenous saline

Figure 9.1 Concentration of the blood in cholera

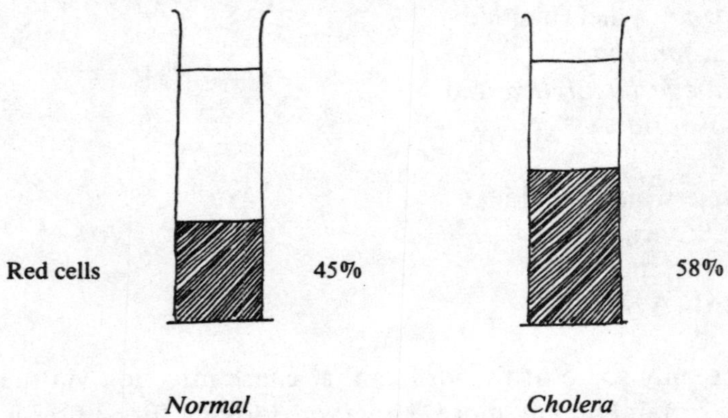

drip; this is impossible in those parts of the world where diarrhoea is most common but fortunately it is possible to replace both salts and water by mouth. A special double-ended spoon has been devised for use by native mothers to measure glucose, salt and bicarbonate. This is dissolved in water and given to the patient. This method of oral replacement should save thousands of lives.

Dysentery

Dysentery is sometimes used as a general term for severe diarrhoea, the cause of which has not been yet discovered. Strictly speaking, it is diarrhoea caused by infection by one of a small family of bacteria (the dysentery organisms) or by an amoeba (*Entamoeba histolytica*). Each of the subfamilies of the bacteria is named after a bacteriologist—a lasting memorial, but in doubtful taste—Shiga (Japanese), Flexner (American), Sonne (Scandinavian) and Boyd (British). The severity of illness of each subfamily is as follows:

Subfamily	*Severity of illness*
Shigella shiga	Severe
Shigella flexner	Intermediate
Shigella boydii	Intermediate
Shigella Sonnei	Mild

Dysentery in tropical countries is often severe, sometimes fatal. In the American Civil War almost 2 million soldiers became infected and there were nearly 45,000 deaths. During the Crimean War ten times as many soldiers died of dysentery as died as a result of Russian actions and in the Boer War five times as many soldiers died from dysentery as were killed by the Boers.

Thirty or forty years ago infection with the more dangerous dysentery organisms, especially Flexner, was not uncommon in Britain; mental hospitals were great repositories of odd pathogens and nearly all types could be found there if the inmates were sampled carefully. Gradually the milder Sonne organism became dominant until today it is practically the only type to be contracted in Britain and even this strain is becoming rarer. Twenty years ago it was the scourge of nursery schools and of establishments for the elderly.

Sonne dysentery is not usually a severe infection and symptoms last only a day or so; however, in young babies or the old and frail it can be dangerous and may even kill. It used to be possible to trace the movements of outbreaks along the lines of communication from town to town and from school to school. Attempts to eradicate the infection from such a school would usually only slow down the progress of the infection and make the whole business last longer; it was usually best to carry on as usual and allow the outbreak to 'burn out' or to pray for the end of term.

Droplet and contact spread of dysentery

Perhaps the most important situation in which diarrhoeal infection may be contracted other than in food occurs in the play school, where numbers of active infants with no sense of civic hygiene are gathered together for several hours each day. Such children are usually susceptible to Sonne dysentery and, when infected, develop fluid stools; by their very nature such stools are more actively infectious than solid stools — they form droplets, splash and are easily smeared over most of the environment. Investigations in such establishments have shown that *Sh. sonnei* may be readily grown from the chain handle, floor, taps and even the seat. Sonne dysentery is one of the few diseases that can be 'caught from a lavatory seat'!

Food poisoning

This archaic term dates from the early days of public health and indicates sudden onset of diarrhoea and/or vomiting as a result of eating some incriminating food. It has more of a legal meaning today, when infection by certain organisms such as the salmonella organisms may be defined as food poisoning while other conditions such as campylobacter infections are not. It is perhaps best to leave this term to the administrators but a list of those organisms generally accepted as causing food poisoning are listed below.

Infection:	Salmonella
	Staphylococci
Toxins:	Cl. welchii
	B. cereus
	Cl. botulinum

Salmonella infections

The normal bowel contains many millions of 'coliform bacilli' living there harmlessly and perhaps doing good in some ways. Both the salmonella and the dysentery organisms resemble closely these coliform organisms, even sharing many of their surface antigens, and there seems no doubt that the more sinister organisms have evolved from the innocent ones. What advantage has accrued from this is difficult to guess; it would have seemed preferable for them to continue enjoying the free food, shelter and heating provided by the host's alimentary canal than to cause so much trouble as to be expelled forcibly in an attack of diarrhoea, although this might provide an efficient way of spread from person to person.

The salmonella group is a large one with well over 1,000 named varieties. They all cause infection in man and/or animals with diarrhoea as a main symptom but a few are able to invade the bloodstream and set up infections elsewhere in the body. In man the typhoid and paratyphoid bacilli are the most likely to do this but in other animals different types have this effect—in mice *S. typhimurium* causes 'mouse typhoid'.

Before the last world war a list of the names of the salmonella types isolated in Britain read like a Baedeker's guide to the country, with *S. eastbourne*, *S. newport*, *S. london* and many other British town names. The exceptions to this were those types that favoured certain animals. We have noted *S. typhimurium* but *S. choleraesuis* was another type which caused 'swine cholera'.

During the war, however, in order to supplement the limited food supplies of Britain, the USA was very generous. Among the many foods sent were spray dried egg and 10 per cent of batches of this commodity contained salmonella. The lower grades were fed to pigs so that these unfortunate animals soon became infected with such exotic organisms as *S. tennessee*, *S. montevideo* and *S. panama*. The better quality dried egg was also eaten by humans.

It was advised that it should be reconstituted in water immediately before cooking. It was the Wise Virgins who thought ahead and reconstituted it the night before for next day's breakfast. Once the dried egg had been mixed with water the salmonella organisms began to multiply, especially in the warm weather; consequently the Wise Virgins developed severe diarrhoea. The Foolish Virgins reconstituted their dried egg at the very last moment, while putting on their make-up before dashing off to work, so that the salmonella and egg were eaten at a stage where there were not sufficient numbers of salmonella organisms to do any harm. There is a moral there somewhere.

Salmonella organisms and food

Many food substances may become contaminated with salmonella organisms. At one time shellfish were a notorious source of infection because of their habit of filtering large volumes of water through their bodies and thus concentrating any bacteria present, perhaps from sewage dumped into the sea; in France, during the period of fifteen years between the world wars, 100,000 cases of typhoid fever, with 25,000 deaths, were ascribed to eating shellfish. Today, however, those shellfish that are eaten raw (and most others) are allowed to 'wash themselves out' in clean water for an adequate period before they are marketed; those that are cooked before being eaten are usually practically sterilized by this process.

Raw meat frequently harbours salmonella organisms. This is due to the high level of salmonella infection in livestock, which has, indeed, been described as being out of control; this is partly because, in the past, much of the fish and bone meal included in animal food and obtained from Asia and South America contained many salmonella organisms.

(It has been possible to find many strange things in consignments of bone meal; an Irish colleague of mine claimed to have found the body of a soldier in full uniform!) Today more care is taken about the treatment of bonemeal before it is incorporated into animal food or garden fertilizer.

A very important factor in the spread of salmonella among livestock today is the large, and mainly unnecessary, amount of travelling that cattle are subjected to before slaughter. This not only lowers the resistance of the animals through stress but ensures that they have every opportunity to become infected and infectious during their travels.

Infected animals produce infected meat which may infect humans directly but infection can also be passed on before slaughter through milk or droppings. Although raw meat is almost always cooked before consumption (with the exception of steak tartare, which should be avoided), it is only too easy to contaminate ready cooked meats, such as ham, tongue and pies, with knives or working surfaces previously used for raw meat.

Three to 4 per cent of sausages and a large proportion of poultry also carry salmonella organisms. About 1 per cent of duck eggs are reported to contain salmonella organisms and as about 100 million duck eggs are used annually in Britain this represents a large number of salmonella organisms. Duck eggs have long been known to constitute a source of salmonella infection because, in many cases, the organism was present in the genital tract so that the eggs were laid with the organisms within the shell. This appears to be happening in the case of hen eggs now, especially in the case of *Salmonella enteritidis* phage type 4, so that these will have to be treated in the same way as duck eggs and be well cooked before consumption. The use of raw hen eggs in mayonnaise and similar dishes and in prairie oysters is to be avoided. Hospital (and other) kitchens must never use shell eggs for uncooked or lightly cooked preparations.

Unpasteurized milk may be contaminated with salmonella organisms by the cow but pasteurized milk is safe unless contaminated afterwards or inadequately treated. The percentage of dogs found to excrete salmonella organisms varies from 1 per cent to 43 per cent so that these animals may cause infection, especially in children. Tinned pet food is sterile but raw horse meat intended for dogs is not more likely to be safe than meat intended for humans.

Sometimes the chain of infection is not obvious. Calves on a farm were carriers of a type of salmonella and the farmer's children contracted the same infection although they had no contact with the calves.

Figure 9.2 A salmonella chain

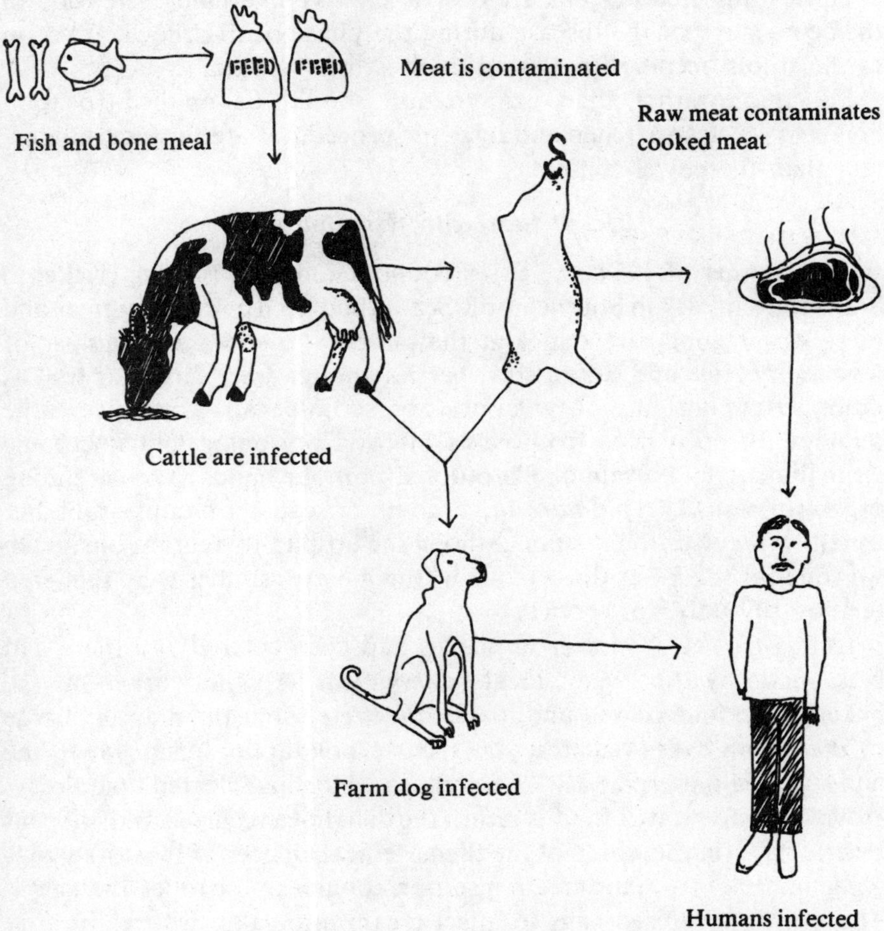

However, the farm dogs wandered everywhere, including the calf pens and the house, and were found to be carrying the strain in question and most probably infected the children. (See Figure 9.2.)

Food handlers

Strangely enough, salmonella infections rarely derive from infected food handlers but usually from food contaminated from the animal. Much stress is laid upon the examination of stools from food handlers by many commercial food manufacturers but this is mostly to impress the customer. Routine specimens are of no value, at least in Western countries; infected persons are only likely to contaminate the food in the acute stage of the disease during the phase of diarrhoea. As soon as the stools become firm again there is little danger.

Education rather than examination should be applied to food handlers. A clean kitchen and hygienic procedures are far more important than the bowel contents.

Cricket teas with typhimurium

In the summer of 1954, the Essex county team were playing cricket in Southchurch Park in Southend-on-Sea. It had been a warm summer and there was a good attendance at the match. There were a number of hospitality tents and cakes, strawberries and tea were served as well as more sustaining fare. My laboratory soon began to receive large numbers of specimens from cases of food poisoning and it became clear that we had a salmonella outbreak on our hands. The offending organism was *S. typhimurium*, a common cause of unpleasant but usually mild infection in man. Among the hospitality tents at the match was one for the Essex doctors, of whom a large number were rendered temporarily unfit for service.

In this particular tent cream cakes had been offered and these had been made by the largest local bakery firm. All the workers at the bakery were interviewed and it was discovered that the man in charge of the cream cakes had recently spent a holiday in Jersey, where he had suffered a sharp attack of diarrhoea which had cleared up quickly. However, a few days after his return the diarrhoea recurred and he spent several days (in the words of the then Medical Officer of Health) 'struggling manfully from the cream insertion counter to the toilet and back!' Those who have used bags to inject cream into cakes will realize that the operation is not possible without considerable involvement of the hands as well.

There were about 400 diagnosed cases in this outbreak and probably about twice as many mild cases who did not go to their doctor.

In Leicester, in the mid 1940s, we had a similar outbreak involving cream cakes. The contamination was eventually traced, again, to the person who inserted the cream. He was a nice lad but, like Jenner's son, 'had a rather defective understanding'. He was removed from the job and no more cases occurred locally. A few months later a similar outbreak occurred in nearby Kettering; when we investigated the bakery the first person we saw was our old friend, obviously something of a specialist, happily introducing cream into the cakes.

Typhoid fever

This infection is caused by the 'Godfather' of the salmonella family, known as *Salmonella typhi*. It is one of the select body of salmonella organisms that are able to penetrate the bowel lining and invade the bloodstream. The other common ones to do this are *S. paratyphi A and B*.

The illness

When taken by mouth the bacteria penetrate the bowel lining and pass into the blood. At this stage there are no symptoms because there are so few bacteria but the latter take refuge in cells in various organs, mainly the liver, where they multiply. After an incubation period of about fourteen days they then pass into the blood stream in large numbers. This is signalled by the onset of the illness, with fever, shivering, headache etc.

Like so many organisms spread by the blood, they cause a rash although only a scanty one, known as 'rose spots'. The organisms also invade the kidneys and can be found in the urine, may be an occasional source of infection.

They also infect what may be described as the tonsils at the other end, Peyer's patches, collections of tonsil-like tissue in the wall of the large bowel. It is here that the chief mischief is perpetrated. During the third week of the illness the typhoid bacteria begin to produce ulcers in the region of the Peyer's patches. This has the effect of causing diarrhoea (which rarely occurs *early* in typhoid). This ulceration may also cause one of two fatal complications:

1. The ulcers may penetrate the bowel, resulting in severe infection of the lining of the abdominal cavity by the organisms normally confined to the interior of the bowel, causing peritonitis. (This is an example of the way that some parts of the body can tolerate many organisms without fear of infection (the interior of the bowel) whereas other areas (the peritoneum) have no resistance at all.)
2. The other complication occurs when the ulcer eats into a large blood vessel causing fatal haemorrhage.

However, these complications are rare today both because typhoid fever is now a rare infection in Britain and because the infection can be controlled by antibiotics before the third week is reached. (See Figures 9.3 and 9.4.)

Figure 9.3 Typhoid infection

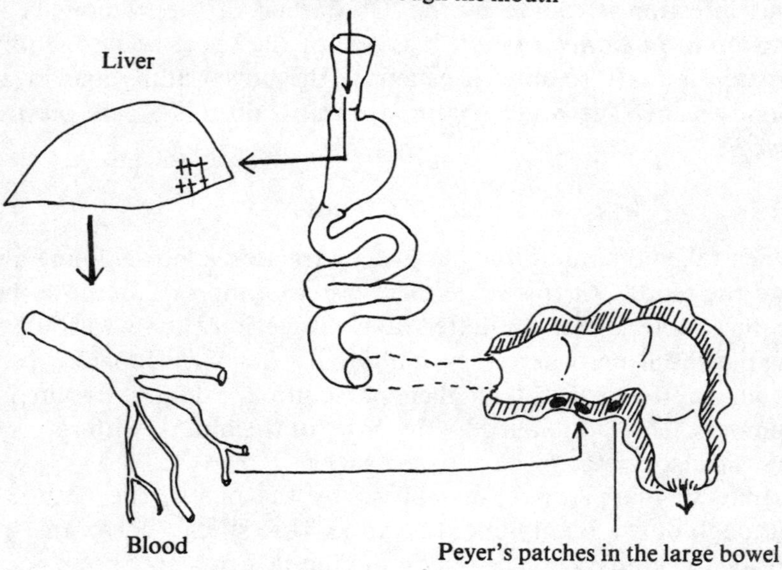

Infection is through the mouth and the typhoid bacilli pass from the bowel to the liver, where they multiply. After about fourteen days they return to the blood and are carried all over the body. Abscesses in Peyer's patches in the wall of the large bowel may result in fatal haemorrhage or perforation.

Contracting typhoid fever

Typhoid fever was only distinguished in the public mind from typhus (an infection spread by rats and lice) in about 1840; both diseases were common in the Britain of that time (typhus was also known as 'gaol fever'). Typhoid often caused huge outbreaks in the nineteenth century, as in Maidstone in Kent where there were 2000 cases among 34,000 inhabitants, and it was said that there were few family doctors in Britain who did not have one or two cases to look after at any one time. Two characteristics of typhoid fever are:

1. Only a few bacteria are needed to cause infection – some workers think one only.
2. After infection, which sometimes is very mild indeed, some patients become carriers and proceed to excrete the organism in their stools or urine for years or for life, like 'Typhoid Mary' (see Chapter 2).

Figure 9.4 Typhoid fever—haemorrhage and perforation

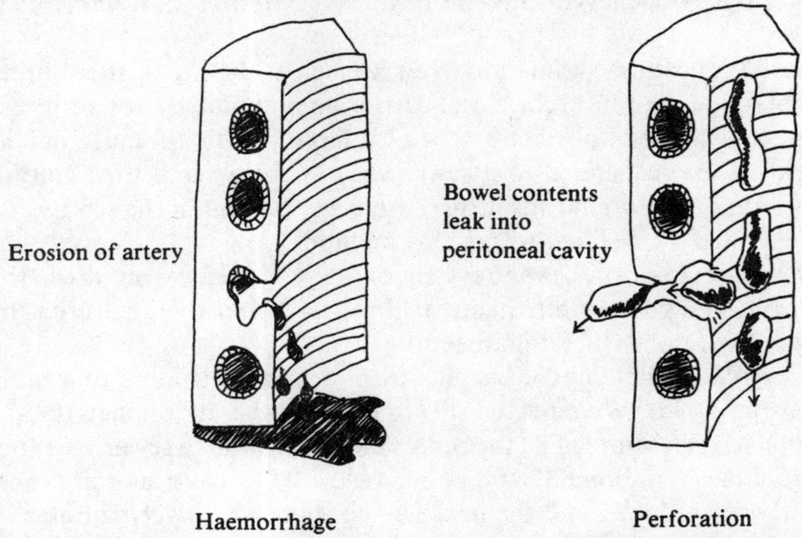

The West Mersea incident

Between 1950 and 1956 twenty cases of typhoid occurred in north Essex. When examined carefully, using a new method, it was found that two different strains of the typhoid bacillus were involved, ten cases being caused by each kind. Lot A were clustered around a lady of sixty-two who had suffered from typhoid sixteen years before and had obviously become a carrier. It was not unusual for ladies in later life to become housekeepers and to begin preparing food for children and grandchildren; several outbreaks of typhoid have occurred when such ladies have been carriers.

When we looked at the other patients whose ages varied between twelve and fifty-one we found the following:

1. Spent one week at West Mersea (early June 1952?).
2. Ate cockles at West Mersea (early August 1952?).
3. Mother and son spent four weeks at West Mersea (October 1952).
4. Ate shellfish in West Mersea (October 1952).
5. Visited West Mersea (October 1953).
6. Patient was in a Colchester hospital from 12 October 1953 but developed typhoid 28 November 1953. Did his visitors bring him oysters instead of grapes?
7. Ate oysters believed to come from West Mersea (December 1953).

8. Ate cockles at West Mersea (July 1955).
9. Ate oysters believed to come from West Mersea (November 1956).

Thus all indications pointed to West Mersea as the site of the source of the infection. But how could the carrier be pinpointed? It had recently been shown that swabs consisting of a large bundle of gauze bandage would, when suspended in a sewer via a manhole and then cultured, grow salmonella organisms if there were any present in the sewage. (See Figure 9.5.) We decided to try this method.

Using a map of the sewage system of West Mersea we put down these swabs at key points, left them for three days and then cultured them in the laboratory. (See Figure 9.6.)

We isolated the typhoid bacillus from a point at the end of a branch sewer (point 30). We repeated this to make sure and obtained the same result and then sampled all the points along the branch sewer. We found typhoid bacilli at point 32 and points below it but never at points above it. Between point 32 and the next one up there were twelve houses. We placed swabs in the inspection chambers of each house and on both the occasions we tested we isolated typhoid bacilli from the chamber of the same house.

The Medical Officer of Health then interviewed the lady who lived there and found that she had suffered a severe attack of typhoid fever in 1948 in what was then Southern Rhodesia and she was found to be still excreting the organism. The lady in question possessed a small sailing boat equipped with a sea-going lavatory. It is possible that she used this at sea and sewage drifted up to the shore.

At that time the oyster fishermen in that part of the world used to place their oysters in pits dug on the foreshore for the dual purposes of storing them and allowing them to cleanse themselves and it is possible that the typhoid bacillus was in the water used for this purpose. A snag in this theory is that two of the patients were infected in December, a season when pleasure sailing was out of the question. A more likely explanation was leakage, in the vicinity of the shore, from the sewage outlet that should have carried the sewage well out to sea but did not.

The lady carrying the typhoid bacillus went on a long holiday and attempts were made, using antibiotics, to cure the carrier state. She returned to West Mersea and in the autumn of 1958 ten further cases occurred, caused by the same strain of the typhoid bacillus but scattered all over England. All had eaten oysters that might have originated from West Mersea about a fortnight before their illnesses. Further

Figure 9.5 Using a 'sewer swab'

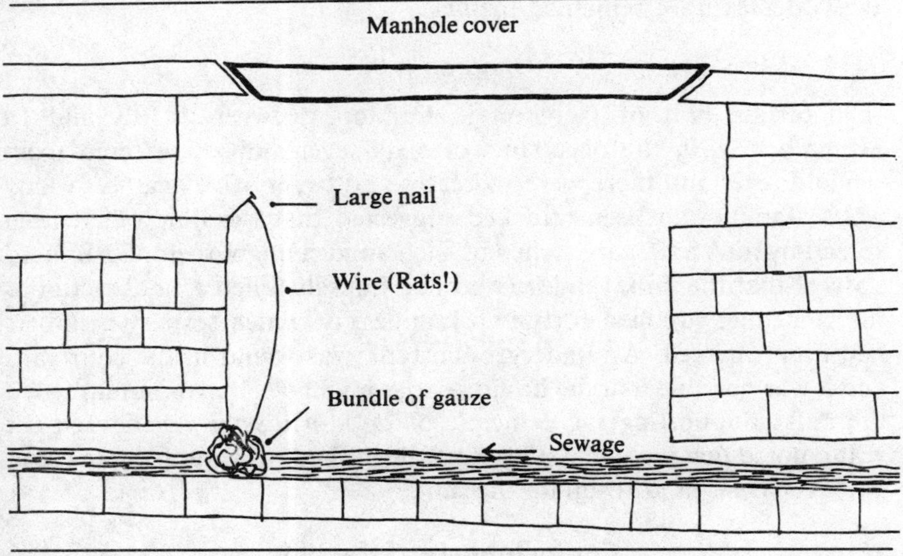

sewer swabs were put down but typhoid bacilli were never isolated from them.

Just at this time the fishermen were beginning to use an improved method of cleaning the oysters by laying them in large tanks of clean water that was sterilized by passage under an ultraviolet lamp (as devised by my friend Peter Wood, later Director of the Ministry of Agriculture,

Figure 9.6 The sewerage system of West Mersea

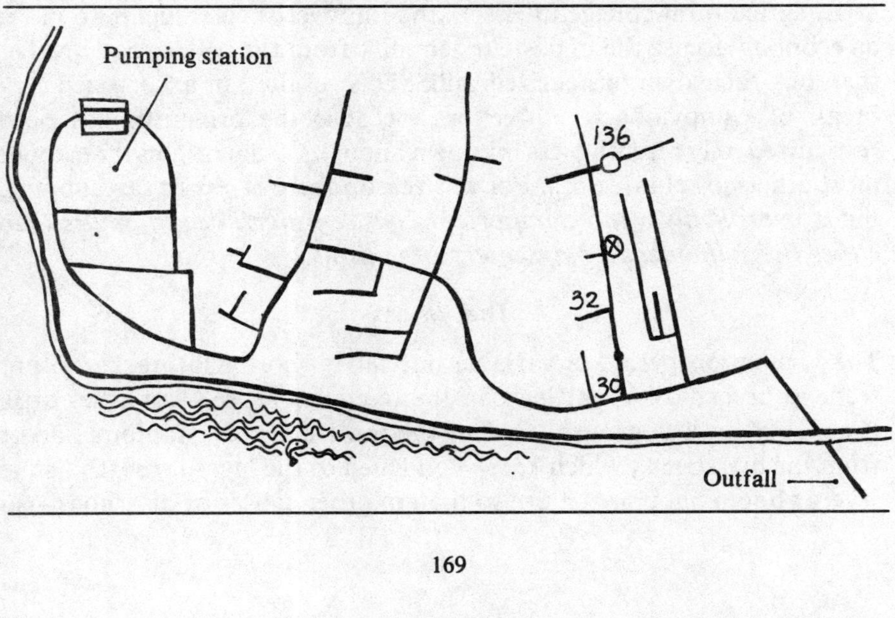

Fisheries and Food laboratory at Burnham). Since then oysters from West Mersea have remained blameless.

Islington milk

In a certain part of Islington in London, between 3 July and 10 September 1870, the occupants of sixty-seven houses suffered from typhoid fever and there were 167 cases and twenty-five deaths. A lady whose family had been attacked suggested that the illness had been spread by milk and, far-fetched as such an idea might seem, Dr Ballard showed that the milk vendor (who had himself fallen a fatal victim to the epidemic) supplied forty-two families, of which seventy members had been infected. An underground tank was found in the courtyard and it was possible that the liquid sewage might well have contaminated the milk. Supporting the principle of *de mortuis nil nisi bonum* the writer noted that it could not be ascertained that the water from the tank had ever been used to dilute the milk!

Campylobacter infection

About 1977 new methods of 'sorting out' various bacteria, especially some short spiral ones, revealed that a large proportion of those bowel infections that could not previously be diagnosed were caused by an organism that was named 'Campylobacter'. This organism is often found in chickens and many outbreaks have occurred both in those handling chickens and also in those eating them.

The organism may also be present in unpasteurized cow's milk and, at an agricultural college in Essex, the impoverished students found it an economy to use the unpasteurized milk from the college cows rather than buy their own pasteurized milk. This resulted in a fair-sized outbreak of campylobacter infection. Because the organism has been recognized only recently, less is known about its usual origins than about most other bowel infectors. For this reason there is less to say about it, but it is *probably a more important cause of diarrhoea in adults than either the salmonella or dysentery organisms.*

The illness

The incubation period is variable but fairly short. Outbreaks do not seem to be explosive – at least in the temporal sense – but cases arise irregularly in little groups. One of the most marked symptoms, apart from the diarrhoea ('which keeps you glued to the lavatory seat'), is the severe abdominal pain – more so than in other causes of diarrhoea – so that some cases are mistakenly taken for surgical emergencies and the patients' normal appendixes removed!

The organism fairly often invades the bloodstream causing fever and shivering attacks. The infection is self-limited but can be cut short with antibiotics.

Food poisoning involving preformed toxins

There are three organisms that can cause diarrhoea and vomiting in this way:

Staphylococcus aureus
Cl. welchii (Cl. perfringens)
Bacillus cereus

There is one other that may cause serious paralysis: *Cl. botulinum*.

Staphylococcus aureus food poisoning

Staphylococci are small round bacteria that cause boils and carbuncles and other skin infections as well as more serious conditions such as bone abscesses. Many normal people carry these organisms in the nose and such people as well as those with tiny skin infections may contaminate food when preparing it. Custards, trifles and meat jellies are fine media for their growth as is also the jelly to be found in the best meat pies.

As we saw, on a warm summer night, one bacterium can become several million in a few hours. (See figures under the heading 'Bowel Infections' in Chapter 2.) During that time sufficient toxin or poison may be produced as to cause severe symptoms. The onset of illness is usually within two hours of eating and vomiting is the main symptom. So much vomiting may take place that the patient collapses through loss of fluid and salts but within a few hours the attack passes and within a few days the patient will have recovered completely. Although unpleasant, the illness does not last long and deaths are very unusual even in frail old people. As the illness is caused by a toxin the patient is not infectious.

Clostridium welchii (clostridium perfringens) food poisoning

Clostridium welchii, now known as *Clostridium perfringens*, is the organism that causes gas gangrene, a condition rarely seen today because of the efficiency of antibiotics. It is normally present in the intestine of animals and man, in dust and on the surfaces of carpets.

It is an anaerobe and cannot multiply in the presence of oxygen. The strains that cause food poisoning are very resistant to heat so that they are capable of multiplying and producing their toxin in the middle of an undercooked joint. This is not a very powerful toxin and causes mild diarrhoea and general internal discomfort. The organism can also survive in the depths of a large vat of gravy where there is no dissolved oxygen so that, when the source of heat is removed, it multiplies and produces toxin as the temperature slowly falls.

In a large Scottish hospital the consultants complained of abdominal discomfort and slight diarrhoea following each occasion there was chicken on the menu in the dining room. The catering officer insisted that everything in the kitchen was as it should be but still the condition grumbled on. One of the laboratory technicians was walking out with a female member of the kitchen staff and he persuaded her to let him into the kitchen at night with his camera (the reasons he gave her for making this visit are not stated). He was able to confront the catering officer with photographs of the offending chickens, not cooled quickly and then refrigerated, but stuffed in quantity into large cooking vessels where they cooled so slowly that *Cl. welchii* had every opportunity to flourish and produce its toxin.

Bacillus cereus food poisoning

This organism became important with the proliferation of Chinese restaurants. Chinese fried rice is usually produced by boiling a large quantity, allowing it to cool and then frying small amounts as required. The mass of rice is not refrigerated and *Bacillus cereus* is fairly heat resistant. It multiplies in the rice and produces its toxin, which is not destroyed by the subsequent frying. Two sorts of food poisoning follow: either vomiting 1 to 5 hours after the meal with minimal diarrhoea, or a more severe diarrhoea coming on between 8 and 14 hours after the meal. The former is more common and both conditions are brief and self-limiting but an unfitting introduction to the pleasures of Oriental food. (This condition is not confined to Oriental restaurants in Britain; I recently suffered it in India.)

Clostridium botulinum food poisoning (botulism)

In 1922 eight sportsmen set out on a fishing expedition on Loch Maree in Scotland. Their catch may have been a good one but in the end wild life had its revenge because within a week they were all dead, poisoned by botulinum toxin in the wild duck paste in their sandwiches.

'Botulinum' means 'to do with sausages' and the organism in question has been found in that item of food. It has three main characteristics: it is heat resistant; it cannot grow in the presence of oxygen; and it produces a very powerful toxin, one milligram being capable of killing approximately 1,200,000 guinea-pigs (were so many available!). It is, fortunately, not a common cause of illness: only five outbreaks have been identified in Britain but the case fatality in outbreaks is very high.

The organisms of the group are not rare and are commonly found in places where oxygen is scarce, as in mud in the floors of estuaries, so that outbreaks of the disease occur quite often among seabirds. It was first discovered in 1896 during a music club festival in Ellezelles in Belgium. As a result of eating a piece of raw ham several players became ill and three died. When some of the remaining ham was given to the cat, it, too, became paralysed and died; the organism was isolated from the ham, the patients and the cat.

Acquiring the illness

As the illness is caused by a toxin there is no spread from affected patients to other people. As the organism thrives in the absence of oxygen it does well in rotting meat where other organisms rapidly use up all the oxygen present.

Some recipes for disaster

Izushi. A Japanese delicacy. Take raw fish, rice and vegetables; soak the fish four to five days, add to the rice and vegetables and allow to ferment for three to four weeks; eat without cooking.

Seal Flippers. An Eskimo dish. Soak seal flippers in seal oil until they rot; then eat raw. Whale flukes, especially when found partly decomposed, may be used in the same way. Whole families of Eskimos have been found dead in their igloos as a result of botulism acquired from such delicacies.

Salmon Egg Cheese. A North American Indian delicacy. Keep salmon eggs in a basket under the bed until they form a sort of cheese.

Ashbai. An Iranian version of the above, using carp eggs.

All the above delicacies have caused death from botulism on many occasions.

In the American Middle West home canning used to be an economic way of putting aside food for the future. Unfortunately, the cans containing the food were heated in water in large saucepans so that the food only just reached boiling point, insufficiently hot to kill the spores of *Cl. botulinum*. As the food cooled the spores multiplied, producing its toxin and behaving as a culinary time-bomb.

One lady canned mushrooms in this way and died after eating some. Her daughter and daughter-in-law opened another tin after their mother's funeral and both, in turn, died after eating some of the mushrooms. *Cl. botulinum* was isolated from all three bodies. If a pressure cooker had been available for use the deaths would not have happened.

In June 1989, a number of patients were admitted to hospitals in northwest England suffering from a variety of neurological illnesses. Many were of the wrong age groups for the illnesses at first suspected and in four instances there were more than one patient in the same family. This led to a suggestion that the outbreak might be due to botulism and this, in fact, was the case. All but two of the patients were discovered to have eaten hazelnut yoghurt in the week before they became ill; botulinum toxin was found in one tin of hazelnut purée (used in making the yoghurt) in the stool of one patient and in two cartons of hazelnut yogurt from patients' homes. In one instance children aged 15 and 13 in one family suffered from the illness after sharing a carton of the yoghurt; the remainder was eaten by the cat who, more fortunate than his Belgian colleague, survived.

In this outbreak only one person out of twenty-seven died. This was probably due to the early recognition of the outbreak; at least two thirds of the affected people were admitted after the earlier cases had been diagnosed so that treatment was commenced at once.

Cholera

This is no longer a disease of any importance in Britain but it was once common and was the stimulus that, from the point of view of public health, dragged us from Third World conditions towards the high standards of today. A few cases occur in Britain most years but these are always contracted abroad. Cholera does not spread from case to case in a developed country and such cases as do occur in Britain are of no public health importance. Prompt treatment involving fluid replacement ensures rapid recovery in almost all cases.

The disease

Cholera is a disease of the Indian subcontinent. On several occasions it has spread far and wide from India and from 1817 onward it has visited Britain on several occasions.

In December 1831 in Sunderland, there were 400 cases in a population of 18,000; 200 people died. In April 1832 in London, there were 11,000 cases, resulting in the deaths of more than 5,000 people. In August of the same year in Bilston (now in the West Midlands), there were 3,500 cases in a population of 15,000; 742 people died. In this first wave, 22,000 died of cholera out of a total population of 14,000,000 in Britain.

In April 1848 in a pauper school at Tooting in London, there were 300 cases in a population of 1,000; 180 people died. Altogether, there were 53,000 deaths in Britain during this outbreak.

In 1853–4, there was a smaller outbreak with about one quarter of the deaths of the previous outbreak.

Investigations into the causes of cholera

In the days of cholera's first visitation, infection was thought to be due to a miasma, an indefinite condition of the air. Bacteria had not yet been discovered but several wiser doctors believed that infection was caused by something passing from an ill patient to a well person (see Chapter 2 and the story of Dr Semmelweiss).

John Snow, a London doctor, was one such person. He was certain that cholera arose by people coming into contact with excreta from cholera patients. He was particularly interested in the Broad Street Pump, a source of water for part of the East End of London; he showed that its water was probably polluted by sewage and he found that far more people who used the water from this pump developed cholera than those who took their water from other sources. An old lady who had moved to the West country asked her daughter to bring her a bottle of water from this pump so that she could taste it before she died. The young lady obliged and the old lady's wish was granted – she died from cholera a few days later. When Snow confiscated the handle of the Broad Street pump, the incidence of cholera in the vicinity declined but the Board of Health did not at first accept Snow's findings, although further discoveries convinced them.

At about this time two companies supplied water to London. In 1849 both were drawing water from the Thames at Westminster – this was also a site where raw sewage was discharged into the river so that many got their own back in a microbiological way of speaking. In about 1850 one of these companies began to draw water from above Teddington, where it had not yet been polluted by London sewage. Soon the deaths from cholera were, for the Teddington firm, 11.3 per 1,000 houses supplied and for the other firm, 57.1, thereby showing the relative purity of water from higher up the river.

When the last wave of cholera to reach Britain arrived in 1866 a main drainage system had been carried out for London and all water came from higher up the Thames, where it was unpolluted.

Cholera today

Cholera is not a serious cause of illness in the Western world but it still causes thousands of deaths in the Third World. It is characteristically a disease of refugees: people herded together in unsanitary and crowded conditions with insufficient medical services; people who use a stream or lake as a source of drinking water and for washing and as a lavatory. Under these conditions cholera spreads rapidly.

A severe case of cholera will pass up to sixty litres of fluid stools ('ricewater stools'), which contain about 100,000,000 organisms per millilitre, so that a patient will pass 6 million million organisms. When such large numbers are concerned it is not surprising that cholera spreads rapidly.

Prevention and management

Cholera is an ever-present danger in the Third World. Most cases of the infection would recover rapidly if sufficient medical services were available to provide rapid intravenous saline drips; but these can only be supplied if the number of cases is small, in view of the relative poverty of the countries where cholera is most common. As a substitute, oral replacement of salt and water seems to be very valuable if the sufferers can be persuaded to use it. A vaccine is available but it is perhaps the least useful vaccine in current use. It is used mainly as an administrative instrument, probably to indicate that the medical authorities of the country where the infection occurs are taking active (but not always useful) steps. If a really effective vaccine could be devised it would be one of the most useful ever produced, in view of the annual death rate from this infection.

Hepatitis A

Hepatitis A is another infection that, although taken in by mouth, produces effects in other parts of the body. We have already discussed hepatitis B, which is spread mainly by homosexual contact. This is not true of hepatitis A, which is always contracted by eating or drinking contaminated food or water.

Figure 9.7 Hepatitis A

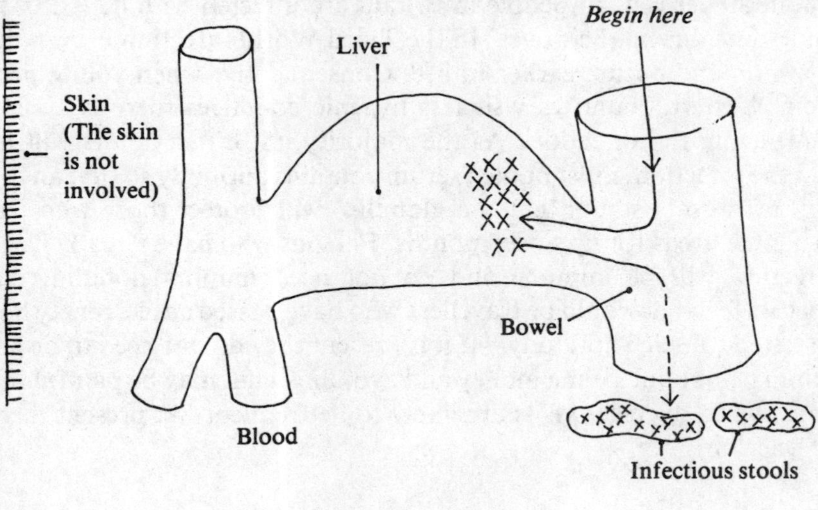

The virus is taken in through the mouth and enters the blood for a short time and then passes to the liver where it causes damage. It multiplies in the bowel and is excreted in the stools which are the source of infection. Compare with Hepatitis type B which enters through the skin, multiplies in the liver and is present in the blood, rendering it infectious often for a long period.

The illness

Hepatitis A is caused by a virus which is not very impressive and simply described as a 'small round virus'. It is usually drunk in contaminated water and it passes through the bowel wall to the blood and thence to the liver. Here it multiplies and after about three to four weeks it has multiplied sufficiently to cause damage to the liver. (See Figure 9.7.) As in infections caused by the hepatitis B virus, this disorganizes the bile tubules and results in the bile pigments being dammed back in the blood, causing jaundice and clay-coloured stools. The infection is not as severe as hepatitis B and death is very rare.

Patients do not become chronic carriers after the infection, although the virus may be present in the stools until the jaundice appears, usually about six weeks after the infection has been contracted. The patient often feels unwell, has a poor appetite for a week or two before the jaundice appears and then rapidly recovers.

Incidence and prevention

About 80 per cent of people in Britain are infected with hepatitis A at some time during their lives. In the Third World infection is even more common and occurs earlier in life. Consequently, when young people from Western countries visit less hygenic countries there is a risk of contracting the infection. As the majority of British adults will have had the infection, most pooled serum contains antibody so that an injection of normal serum (gamma globulin) will protect those who travel to danger areas for up to six months. Persons who have already had the infection will be immune and do not need immunoglobulin; many doctors feel that would be travellers who have passed adolescence should be tested for such antibody – if it is present they do not need to be given gamma globulin, saving money and avoiding what may be painful injections, when overseas visits are likely to be frequent. At present there is no vaccine.

Amoebic dysentery

We have already discussed the type of dysentery caused by bacteria. There is another sort, occurring mainly in the tropics, caused by an amoeba, *Entamoeba histolytica*. 'Histolytica' means capable of destroying tissues, a reference to the fact that the amoeba buries itself in the lining of the bowel.

The disease

The patient suffers from severe diarrhoea and abdominal pain. The condition resembles ulcerative colitis very closely and, in the latter condition, it is sometimes necessary to remove the colon, leaving an unpleasant permanent condition. Amoebic dysentery is not common in Britain, where a few cases have been misdiagnosed and the patient's colon removed unnecessarily. I have seen two cases practically snatched from the surgeon's knife at the last moment by finding amoebae in material removed from the bowel by biopsy. Thus, all cases diagnosed as ulcerative colitis should be investigated for the presence of *Entamoeba histolytica* and even treated as amoebic dysentery with the appropriate drugs before surgery, just in case. The infection responds very promptly to the drug metranizadole.

The disease is contracted by eating food contaminated with cysts, usually from infected food handlers. Within the small intestine the cysts break down; this releases the amoebae, which multiply and pass to the large bowel where they tunnel into the lining, causing haemorrhage and inflammation.

Occasionally, the amoebae penetrate the wall of a blood vessel and are carried to the liver, where they cause an abscess to form; as there is some disorganization of the bile tubules (as in virus hepatitis, but less severe) a mild jaundice occurs which may last a long time. Old campaigners from India frequently complained of an irritable bowel and a touch of jaundice—'a touch of liver, old boy, as Major Bloodnock of 'The Goon Show' would have said.

The spread of amoebic dysentery

Spread occurs through food handlers who are excreting the cysts. In the Third World it might be appropriate to screen such workers regularly but, in the West, this is needed only after an attack of diarrhoea. In 1933 in Chicago, an incompetent plumber connected the sewage systems of two hotels to the water supply and caused 1,400 cases and over 100 deaths.

The disease is rare in Britain but should be suspected in patients with chronic diarrhoea, especially if they have been abroad for any length of time.

Cryptosporidiosis

The cryptosporidium is a single celled parasite related to the toxoplasma discussed in Chapter 4. During the 1960s and 1970s veterinary workers discovered that the cryptosporidia caused some cases of animal diarrhoea. Such infected animals can infect man and, since 1976, a large number of human cases and outbreaks have been observed.

Outbreaks have occurred in nurseries, families and hospitals (where staff have been infected by patients). The organism has sometimes been found in association with another single cell cause of diarrhoea, *Giardia lamblia*, and the two have been found together in water supplies. Cryptosporidium first achieved public notoriety when a water authority recommended that its water should be boiled before being given to young children because of the possible presence of cryptosporidium.

Diarrhoea lasts up to fourteen days but attacks are usually mild and need no treatment. The condition seems to be nearly as common as rotavirus infection in young children.

Virus infections

The viruses that cause gastroenteritis are not very exciting, resembling those causing hepatitis A, but they may be responsible for more intestinal infections than all the other causes put together. Most of the illnesses they cause are mild.

Rotaviruses

This group of viruses affects both man and animals but the animal types do not infect man and vice versa. For years the causes of most outbreaks of diarrhoea in children in hospitals and other institutions remained a mystery; but toward the end of the 1970s it was found that, if the stools from these patients were examined under an electron microscope, many contained large numbers of viruses with wheel-like markings. Such viruses were already known to cause diarrhoea in animals and it was soon established that most infections in children were caused by similar ones. Recently a vaccine prepared by growing monkey types of rotavirus in tissue culture have been shown to protect over 90 per cent of babies from 1 to 5 months old against the infection.

The illness

Children between the ages of six months and four years are affected. The incubation period lasts two to three days, followed by the passage of loose yellow-green offensive stools. It is probable that the infection comes from the children's attendants.

The illness is mild and short-lived and there is no specific treatment; solid food may be omitted for a time but drinking should be encouraged. The virus also affects elderly people and outbreaks in old persons' homes have been recorded.

The Norwalk group

There are a number of similar viruses called simply 'small round viruses' that can cause gastroenteritis. Unlike the rotaviruses, all ages may be infected and nausea and vomiting are commoner than diarrhoea. Outbreaks may occur in families or in institutions following ingestion of contaminated food or water; it is likely that many cases of gastroenteritis following bathing in contaminated seawater or eating shellfish taken from such water are caused by this group of viruses. A typical outbreak occurred in Colchester following a dinner where 'prawn cocktail' was replaced by 'seafood cocktail', consisting of pieces of cockle in cocktail sauce. About a day later a large proportion of those eating this cocktail developed sickness, in many cases followed by diarrhoea. Similar illness in two of the children of a patient a day or two later indicated that this was an infectious condition and not caused by a poison or a bacterial toxin.

Illness caused by the Norwalk group of viruses is always mild. Because of the difficulty in identifying the virus (even in outbreaks), the real cause is not usually found and, every year, thousands of sporadic cases must occur that are never investigated.

TEN

The Arthropods

The arthropods can injure humans in two different ways: primarily, by acting as transfer agents (vectors) in spreading infection from person to person or from animal to human and, secondarily, as sources of injury and annoyance in their own right.

Arthropods as vectors of infection

In many instances man is an accidental victim of an infection which is usually confined to animals but is contracted 'in error' when he happens to be bitten by the arthropod that normally spreads the infection from animal to animal. An example is sylvatic yellow fever, where mosquitoes transfer the virus usually from monkey to monkey; a man in the wrong place at the wrong time may be bitten by the mosquito and may share the monkey's infection.

The following infections may be contracted as a result of arthropod bites.

Organisms	*Diseases caused*	*Vectors*
Plague bacilli	Plague	Rat fleas
Rickettsiae	Typhus	Rat fleas Body or head lice Ticks
Borrelia burgdorfia	Lyme disease	Ticks
Malarial parasites	Malaria	Mosquitoes
Trypanosomes	Sleeping sickness	Tsetse flies
Trypanosomes	South American trypanosomiasis	Reduviid bugs
Leishmania	Leishmaniasis (Tropical ulcer)	Sandflies

Arboviruses	Various including yellow fever	Mosquitoes Sandflies Ticks
Filaria (Tiny worms)	Filariasis (Elephantiasis)	Mosquitoes Midges Black flies Deer flies

In many cases the offending organisms merely multiply in the arthropod vector; in the case of typhus the rickettsiae (small bacterium-like bodies that cannot be grown on artificial medium) do so and are excreted in the faeces and the victim obligingly scratches these into the bite.

The plague bacillus multiplies so abundantly in the vicinity of the stomach of the flea that a blockage is caused. Efforts on the part of the flea to suck up blood result in the flea regurgitating blood into the bite together with plague bacilli.

The above organisms undergo little change within their arthropod vectors but most parasites not only multiply but also undergo changes in form within the vector. The malarial parasite, for instance, enjoys sexual reproduction only in the mosquito and not in man. This procedure usually means that a period within an arthropod is needed before the organism can become infective; it also means that the arthropod is *not* infective immediately after becoming infected (by taking blood from an infected man or animal) but only after a period of time, which may be days or weeks and depends to some extent on the atmospheric temperature.

The arboviruses

The viruses carried by arthropods are so numerous that they have been described as 'arboviruses', which is short for 'arthropod-borne viruses'. There are about 500 types, of which over eighty affect man. The best known are those causing yellow fever and dengue.

Arthropods annoying in their own right

As the insect vectors involved in causing infection will usually be described when talking about the individual infecting organisms, the remainder of this chapter is devoted to arthropods that are in themselves nuisances to man. They include:

Insects	Lice
	Fleas
	Bedbugs
	Flies (including mosquitoes)
Mites	The Scabies Mite
Ticks	

Lice

There are three types of lice that infect man: the crab louse, the body louse and the head louse. (See Figure 10.1.)

Lice feed only on blood so that, with a population of several hundred lice feeding five to six times a day and injecting their saliva into the blood at each feed, it is not surprising that their host feels weary, irritable and

Figure 10.1 Lice

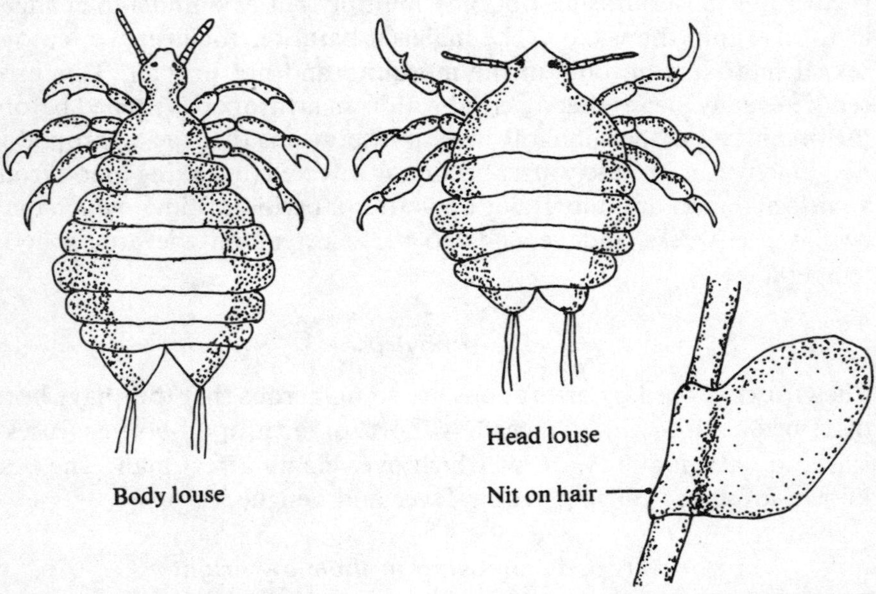

pessimistic. As the book says: 'The lousy feel lousy!' Prolonged biting leads to scratching which causes secondary infection. With severe infestation large amounts of louse faeces may be produced; this may appear as a black powder which causes a sort of 'hay fever' if inhaled by a sensitized person. Lice are also vectors for carrying typhus and relapsing fever – fortunately not common diseases in the West.

Crab lice

This strain prefers widely spaced coarse hair so that it lives in the pubic region, although it may also affect hairy legs and underarm hair and may even be found in beards. It is about 1.5 mm long and difficult to see. It takes about three weeks from infection to the appearance of symptoms; so that a sufferer might blame the public lavatory seat of a week ago rather than his bedmate of three weeks before. For self-medication modern veterinary flea powders are effective but flysprays, paraffin and petrol are not (and the last two may cause a severe and painful conflagration!). A medical lotion containing gamma benzene hydrochloride may be used and should be allowed to act for six hours.

Body lice

Body lice do not live on the body but in the clothing, especially the seams. A cartoon from the First World War shows a tommy running a lighted candle along the seam of his vest. He explains that he is 'toasting the visitors'. The louse lives in the seams of the clothing and ventures out at mealtimes to feed at the skin surface.

Eggs hatch in seven days and the young lice must drink blood within 36 hours, after which they mature in a further seven days. The lice live in the clothing and when this is removed from the patient the lice are also removed. The condition may be suspected if the bites follow where the seams of the underclothes would have been. Bitten areas, after a time, become permanently stained – a condition known as 'Vagabond's disease'.

Lice will not move in bright light, and, when dealing with lousy clothing, the only precaution necessary is to prevent one's own clothing from touching it. Clothes can be deloused by putting them into a tumble dryer for five minutes. There is no need to treat the patient, only his clothes.

Head lice

Head lice are an ancient nuisance: nits have been found in the locks of an Egyptian mummy and also in the mummy of an American Indian of over 4000 years ago. This louse is 2–4 mm long and has a lifespan of thirty days. The female lays 6–8 eggs per day and glues them to a hair and they hatch in seven days. The young louse (nymph) becomes adult in a further ten days but the egg case (the 'nit') remains stuck to the hair and is carried away from the scalp as the hair grows; hence, any nits more than about 1 cm from the scalp will be empty. Lice need warmth and deviations in the patient's temperature from 37°C, as in high fever or death, will cause them to leave the patient as the rat is said to leave the sinking ship. The louse lives in an almost perfect environment and will not move willingly so that infection of new patients demands a close contact of heads, exactly as happens in schools.

Hats, combs, hairbrushes, furniture and seats in theatres and trains play no part in the dissemination of lice. (Some US authorities recommend sterilization of all personal clothing, bedclothes and bedding, disinfection of combs and brushes and the changing of undergarments and night clothes daily; all this is quite unnecessary.)

Head lice have always been common in Britain and in 1940 a survey showed that girls were more likely to be affected than boys; that preschool children were most affected; that boys were less likely to be affected after they passed three years of age, while the girls were still infected in their teens; and that old people were not more likely to be infected than others. The overall infection rate then was about 30 per cent.

There was another increase in the incidence of head lice in the 70s and it was shown in Teesside that, while the incidence of children infected in surburbia was only 0.6 per cent, in downtown areas it was 23 per cent, showing that it is less common in affluent society.

Treatment involves the use of lotions containing malathion or carbaryl. The lotion is rubbed into the hair without washing it and the hair is allowed to dry naturally. The hair can be washed 12 to 24 hours later. Toothcombing has no effect on the infection but appears to provide a degree of satisfaction to some school nurses. Shampoos may be used instead of lotions and it is a good idea to treat the whole family at the same time.

Fleas

Fleas have no wings but they can jump great distances and, unlike lice, they do not hesitate to move from host to host. (See Figure 10.2.) They have certain preferred hosts but, lacking their favorite subject, they are willing to make do with a substitute. They are more associated with nests and burrows than with the actual body, either of an animal or a human.

Human fleas

The human flea is known, for obvious reasons, as *Pulex irritans*. The advent of dryer, warmer and cleaner houses has rendered this a candidate for conservation because it prefers dirt and is driven by cold to share more intimately the environment of the human body. Both the flea and its larva live in human beds, especially those with unwashed sheets and blankets. It can breed in the cracks in dirty floors and can use dogs and cats when pushed. Flea bites are usually easily recognizable.

Cat fleas

Today, the cat flea is the most important flea from the human point of view; it is also the commonest flea on the dog. There are always more

Figure 10.2 A flea

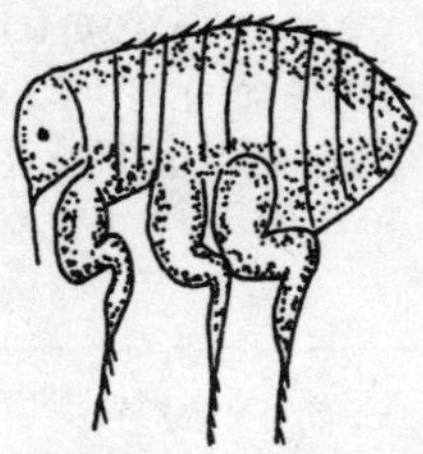

Note the powerful hind legs

fleas *off* the cat than *on* it: for twenty-five fleas on the cat there may be ten times as many in the environment and many more eggs and larvae in the cat litter, etc. Fleas are an infestation of a place rather than a host.

The cat flea may also carry the cyst stage of the dog tapeworm, which can infect children, but with little harm to them. Cat fleas will attack man if he enters the cat's environment and will typically bite the wrists, hands and ankles. Children who have their pets in bed may be bitten on the trunk, sometimes appearing as if they are suffering from an infectious rash.

Rat fleas

The rat flea can carry the plague bacillus and it infects only the black rat, not the brown one. The subject is discussed further in Chapter 13.

Bird fleas

Pigeons, housemartins and a number of other birds have their own peculiar fleas. As with other types of flea, these fleas occupy the nests rather than the birds themselves. When the martins migrate in the autumn, the fleas that are left in the nest look for other hosts and may invade the roof space or even bedrooms, where they may bite the human occupants.

Bed bugs

Bed bugs are about 5 mm in length, flat and oval, possessing no wings. (See Figure 10.3.) They are also known as 'wall lice' because they live in cracks in the walls, from which they venture forth about two hours before dawn to feed on the blood of unconscious sleepers. Bites are usually on the exposed head, hand and arms and the bug voids liquid urine from its anus making small brown stains on the sheets.

Bed bugs can be moved from one house to another in infected furniture. If cracks in suspected walls are sprayed with ordinary flyspray this will irritate the bugs so that they emerge, but it will not kill them. For

Figure 10.3 A bed bug

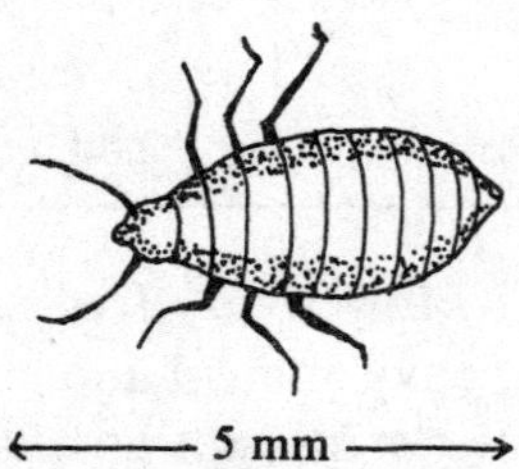

the latter purpose a persistent insecticide, together with redecoration and filling of cracks, is needed. As the bug will not feed at temperatures below 10°C, it is active in the winter months only in houses with central heating.

Superficially similar to the bed lice are the reduviid bugs of South America, the vector for South American trypanosomiasis. (See Figure 10.4.)

Flies

As we shall see, flies may be dangerous carriers of disease, especially in the tropics, where they may carry the parasite that causes sleeping sickness and the minute larval forms of the worms that cause elephantiasis. In addition, some flies can infest man directly.

Figure 10.4 A redurid bug

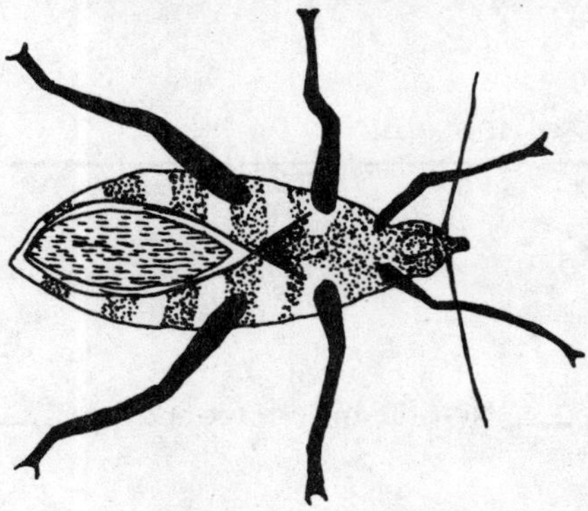

The vector of American trypanosomiasis

Warble flies

The warble fly mainly affects cattle. Its eggs are laid in their hair and, when the grubs emerge, they penetrate the skin and wander all over the cow's body for nearly a year. They then work their way upwards to surface on the cow's back, where a swelling appears which breaks to release the larval form of the fly. This falls to the ground where the rest of the development of the fly takes place.

Occasionally man is infected with a similar course of events, the passage of the grubs through the viscera being very painful. However, when the time comes to leave, the grub, ignorant of the fact that it is in a man (an animal whose back is not normally horizontal), works its way upwards to reach not the back, but the brain, where it may cause severe illness or death.

There are a number of other flies, mostly tropical, that have a predilection for laying their eggs in wounds or other inconvenient places.

My textbook mentions the ingestion of butterfly larvae in uncooked food, a condition called 'scolechiasis'; it remarks that records are rare because the condition (and the butterfly) must usually pass unnoticed.

Mosquitoes

Mosquitoes also belong to the fly family but are sufficiently distinct as to be discussed separately. They act as vectors for a number of parasites, including those that cause malaria, filariasis, yellow fever and encephalitis. (See Figure 10.5.) They do little direct harm but their bites may produce a painful lump in sensitized people a few hours or days after being bitten. Scratching may produce an ulcer and secondary infection may follow.

Figure 10.5 Types of mosquito

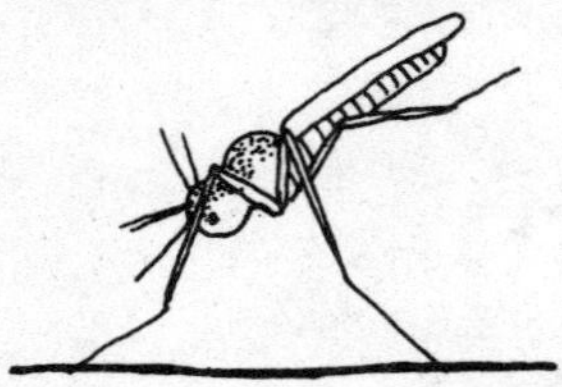

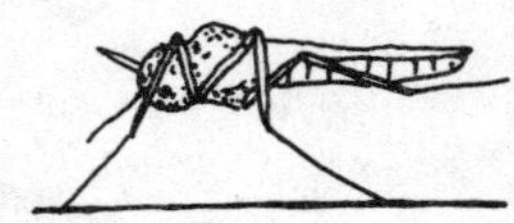

Anopheline

Transmits malaria

Culicine

Transmits arboviruses and filaria but not malaria

Houseflies

Houseflies, together with bluebottles, horseflies, stable flies and others, have been accused of carrying the organisms of dysentery and enteric organisms as well as the virus of poliomyelitis. There is not a lot of evidence for this and, even if it is true, present methods of sewage disposal in Britain must render the risk of contracting disease from these insects very rare indeed.

Scabies

Scabies is an infestation of great antiquity, hallowed by the seal of sanctity by the good saints who took pride in the humility of dirt. It is caused by a mite about 0.5 mm in size. The female burrows within the skin at a rate of 2.5 cm per minute, using her jaws and two front legs. It takes her about fifteen minutes to make the burrow and she remains there for the rest of her life. She lays two eggs each day for one to two months. Adult males make smaller burrows and leave them for a sole purpose: to copulate with the female, which they do once only. There is an interval of fourteen days from the egg to the adult mite. Scabies mites do not suck blood; their very presence in the skin causes severe irritation, most noticeably in subjects especially sensitive to their presence. (See Figure 10.6.)

The spread of scabies is usually by close contact, body to body, and not by dirty bedclothes. However, there is a variety called crusted or Norwegian scabies in which the patient sheds skin scales containing the mites. This variety is very infectious as is suggested by the following outbreak.

Figure 10.6 The scabies mite

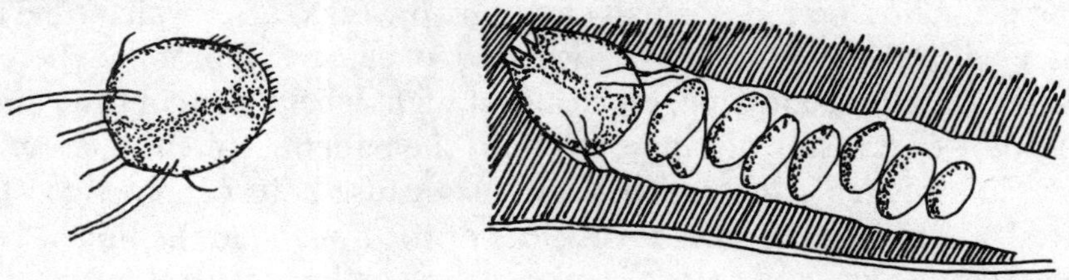

An adult

A female with eggs in a skin burrow

Scabies in the south-west

In 1984 an eighty-one-year-old lady was admitted to a small hospital in the south-west of Britain. She was suffering from what was first thought to be psoriasis, a skin condition that is *not* caused by infection, but two weeks after her admission it was shown to be crusted scabies. By this time several of the staff had itchy rashes and so much concern was felt that, a month after the patient's admission, all persons who had been concerned were invited to the hospital in order to discover the state of play.

Out of forty-three members of staff, twenty were infected as were also members of the families of six nurses and seven auxillaries. The roll call of the affected included:

1 sister
5 staff nurses
1 enrolled nurse
11 auxillaries
the District Nurse
5 husbands
6 children
2 grandchildren
1 porter

This illustrates how extensively and rapidly this type of scabies can spread. In one of the above cases the incubation period was only two days. All the nursing personnel had had close bodily contact with the old lady from time to time, as when lifting her. Another important fact was that several lots of treatment were needed to clear the old lady of her infestation.

The disease

The incubation period is usually about two weeks, after which time the mites will have multiplied sufficiently to cause symptoms. There is usually widespread itching, especially at night when warm in bed. There is also often a rash with tiny blisters; if the patient scratches, infection by organisms from the patients skin may cause boils or impetigo. The mites' burrows can be seen at the sides of the fingers, in the finger webs and on the wrists and soles as tiny wavy black lines several millimetres long. With care the mite may be prised out and identified, using a fine needle rendered sticky with a little mineral oil.

It is fairly important to diagnose the condition in this way, especially in the attendants of a patient with scabies, because itching in one person can, psychologically, generate itching in another and scratching can cause a rash that may be mistaken for scabies. False scabies and fear of scabies (acarophobia) are not uncommon.

Treatment of scabies

Benzoyl benzoate has been the standard treatment for many years and remains so. *When a patient with scabies is treated every member of the household should be treated at the same time as well*. The itching may take some time to disappear after treatment, which may be repeated only with caution, because it may rarely cause dermatitis.

Scabies has its 'waves'; there was an increase in the First World War and another beginning before the Second World War, reaching a peak in 1957. Since 1971 it has reached epidemic dimensions in the USA.

Ticks

Ticks are similar to mites but rather larger. A large number of different infections may be carried by ticks, including relapsing fever. This occurs mainly in Asia and is seldom severe. The causative organism is a loosely coiled spirochoete, *Borrelia duttoni*. After a short incubation period the patient develops a fever lasting a few days; a few days after the temperature has settled another attack occurs. Usually there are three or four episodes before the patient recovers.

Lyme disease

This condition was first described in Old Lyme, Connecticut, USA. Although it is caused by a spirochoete (*Borellia burgdorfia*) carried by a tick (*Ixodes ricinus* in Britain) and is not due to the efforts of the arthropod alone, this seems the most suitable place to discuss Lyme disease. This tick is present in heath and woodland, where it sits on the summits of heather and tufts of grass, waiting for bare knees to pass. These it bites and transfers the spirochoete to the human.

The disease begins with a small spot where the bite occurred, followed by a characteristic rash (*Erythema chronica migrans*) with a fever and sometimes meningitis. The condition may be treated with suitable antibiotics.

About seventy cases have been recognized in Britain in two years but the real number of infections must be much greater as the symptoms may be mild or even absent. A survey of foresters, farmers and gamekeepers in Scotland showed that 12 per cent possessed antibody to *Bor. burgdorfia* in their blood.

ELEVEN

A Trip to the Tropics I

The Industrial Revolution and the origins of public health

Some time during the eighteenth century a change began to take place in the ways that things were made or transported in Britain and other countries of Northern Europe. The basic change was a move away from the use of human (or animal) muscle power toward the use of machines driven by fossil fuel—at first coal, later oil and natural gas and we can perhaps stretch a point and include radioactive substances that are used to provide nuclear fuel.

This primary change brought several secondary changes in its wake. For instance, it was not practical to provide large numbers of small machines so that manufacturing had now to take place at a central place where the necessary machines were sited; in this way factory manufacture replaced the former cottage industries.

This meant that workers began to move from the countryside to the towns in order to find employment in the new factories. The results of this movement involved a great shortage of decent housing and a vast increase in the incidence of infection, due both to the crowding together of large numbers of people and to the terrible conditions under which the poor lived.

The economic effect of the Industrial Revolution was to increase productivity by factors of between 100 and 1,000. Thus, although the majority of citizens were poor, the nations, as entities, became rich. However, some wiser men, having been shown the mechanisms by which certain infections spread (notably with reference to cholera and its spread by drinking water) decided that at least some of the money gained through the Industrial Revolution could be used to mitigate some of the harm it had caused; they recognized, in fact, that money could be used to buy the health of the people and, in this way, the concept of public health began.

The first steps were to provide a safe supply of water for domestic use and an efficient system for the disposal of sewage; this was carried out in time to abort the last important visit of cholera to Britain. Later achievements were the development and—deplorably delayed—introduction of vaccination against infection; the maintenance of safety standards for food; the pasteurization of milk (a hotly debated subject for many years); the ensurance of adequate food intake for all (brought about by food rationing during the Second World War); and, finally, the National Health Service, a much maligned but highly successful basic health system.

Thus, the Industrial Revolution indirectly and in due course gave rise to a culture in which good health became almost the right of all members of the community, whether poor or rich. This is a concept that we, as members of that culture, have grown up with so that we find it difficult to go back two or three centuries and discover, in the Third World, cultures that, from a public health point of view, are those that were current in Britain during the Middle Ages.

In some countries the philosophy of the citizen's absolute right to perfect health seems to have gone too far and immortality seems to be regarded as every man's right; hence, death can only be regarded as an example of medical incompetence.

Infection in the Third World

The enormous burden of infection suffered by citizens of the Third World is almost entirely due to poverty—no Industrial Revolution has occurred there and most industrial methods used are fairly primitive (except in institutions organized by and run for the benefit of members of the developed countries). As an example, I remember a fairly well-educated black Kenyan who was a laboratory technician saying that he measured land by the time it took to walk round it.

A further important factor, in Africa at least, is the complete disorganization in many countries, especially following the granting of independence, by constant bloody quarrels due to tribalism and a general lack of civil conscience.

Infectious diseases in the Third World

We often tend to think that the Third World has special problems because of the warm conditions that prevail in the Tropics. This is partly true in that there are certain diseases (e.g. malaria) which depend for their continued existence on such insects as mosquitoes which, because of the warmer conditions prevailing, are able to enjoy longer personal lives and thus give rise to more infections; however, it should be remembered that malaria was quite common in Britain during the nineteenth century. Nevertheless, such infections could be wiped out or at least greatly reduced if, for instance, there was sufficient money for clearing the areas where mosquitoes breed and for research on the production of a vaccine that might wipe out malaria completely; however, it should also be pointed that we in the West are not in a position to cast stones when measles, whooping cough and rubella, which are eminently preventable diseases in a wealthy culture, still cause widespread illness and death.

Western infections in the Third World

The best-known tropical diseases are those caused by parasites – either the small single-celled ones, such as the malaria organisms, or the larger 'worms'. However, viral and bacterial diseases that were once common in the West are still more common in the Third World. We have seen that poliomyelitis is still common in Brazil; it is probably commoner still in Africa and the Middle East. It has recently been estimated that about 300,000 cases of poliomyelitis occur in the Third World annually; if this is true it is likely that twice this number of young children die undiagnosed from this disease, becoming merely statistics in a high infant mortality rate. Meningococcal meningitis, of which 400–800 cases occur in Britain annually, is responsible for thousands of deaths annually in Africa south of the Sahara. A recent investigation into the causes of a raised temperature in children in a town in Rwanda found that forty-seven out of a total of 900 tested had *Salmonella typhi* in their blood and another thirty-six had other types of salmonella. As the population of the whole of Rwanda is about that of Yorkshire, the comparative number of cases of typhoid fever *in children alone* is enormous compared with the incidence of this disease in Britain.

Viruses out of Africa

The whole of the Third World must be regarded as a huge microbiological laboratory where experiments are carrying themselves out continuously, largely because of its teeming animal life and because poverty brings the people into intimate contact with animal life. The vast majority of these experiments are, from an academic point of view, unsuccessful but a few bring about startling and serious outbreaks of infection.

There are two types of 'experiment' that occur. One is the modification of organisms so that they become more effective in infecting man and the second is constant introduction of animal viruses to man.

To illustrate the first kind of 'experiment', we need only think about influenza A infection. We have already seen that this virus is not of great importance once it has infected a large proportion of the population unless it can change the chemical make-up of its surface, that is, becoming a new type. It is probably not a coincidence that many new types of influenza A seem to have originated in Asia (for instance 'Asian flu' and 'Hong Kong flu'). In this part of the world man and his animals live in close contact and may frequently exchange organisms. It has been shown many times in the laboratory that, when two different varieties of the same virus grow in the same cell, the offspring will frequently show characteristics of both 'parent' viruses. Thus, it is not impossible that the farmer's influenza A virus might co-infect a cell (either in the farmer's lung or that of one of his animals) with an animal strain of influenza A.

If the offspring bear the traits of both 'parents' then we can expect strains of influenza A which, like the parental human strain, can infect and cause illness in man but, because it has the surface constitution of the animal virus, it is not killed by antibody to the parental human strain. Thus the world is now its oyster!

New African viruses

During the Middle Ages, epidemics of plague commonly occurred in the countries of Europe. This disease was spread by rats through their infected fleas and the outbreaks occurred because rats infested practically all human habitations at that time. Now that rats are no longer respectable, plague has disappeared from the Western world, the last outbreak in England occurring in Suffolk just before the First World War. This occurred among people living in rat-infested houses. Once the rats had been removed from the houses no more infections occurred among humans although the bacterium responsible was present in rats and hares in the wild in the neighbourhood. (See Chapter 13.)

In Africa conditions resemble those that occurred in Europe during the Middle Ages. Man lives cheek by jowl with his animals, both wild and domesticated, so that it is not surprising when an organism usually concerned with infecting animals tries its hand at infecting man. These are usually the unsuccessful 'experiments' but on at least three occasions the 'experiments' have been successful from the point of view of the virus concerned.

The viruses concerned were those that cause Marburg disease (green monkey disease), Ebola fever and Lassa fever.

Green monkey disease (Marburg fever)

In 1967 there was an outbreak of serious illness among people associated with a biological institution in Marburg in Germany and also one in Yugoslavia. In all there were thirty-one cases and seven deaths. The illness was characterized by widespread bleeding – into the intestines, the lungs and the skin. One man recovered from the infection but infected his wife some eighty-three days after the onset of his illness. It was found that he was carrying the virus in his semen!

It was shown that the condition was an infection caused by an unusual type of virus which appeared thread-like under the electron microscope.

The outbreak followed the introduction into the biological institute of a batch of green monkeys from Uganda and these monkeys were found to be harbouring the virus. Investigation of other green monkeys both in other laboratories and in the wild failed to yield the virus responsible for the outbreak.

Eight years later a couple hitch-hiked and walked through Rhodesia and part of South Africa. The man became ill and died in hospital in South Africa from Marburg virus infection. His companion was infected but recovered, while a nurse who had tended him in hospital and who developed the infection also recovered.

Lassa fever

Outbreaks of this disease have occurred in Nigeria, in Sierra Leone and in Liberia. The first outbreak occurred in Lassa in Northern Nigeria in 1969. The virus is a round virus distantly related to the rubella virus.

The first victim was a mission nurse who may have been infected by a patient not known to have the disease. She was transferred to a larger hospital but died. One of the nurses who cared for her became ill and died, then the senior nurse became ill. She was flown back to the USA in the first-class cabin of a scheduled airliner, with only a curtain separating her from other passengers! There were, fortunately, no infections contracted on the flight. A virologist who had dealt with material from the last case became ill but recovered slowly after being given serum from the case he had dealt with. Five months later a technician in the same laboratory, who had never worked with the virus or with material from patients infected with it, contracted the infection and died; the source of his infection was never discovered.

The virus is present in rodents known as multimammate mice which may live in the wild or in houses of the local people. It can be isolated from these animals and they seem to be the source of most sporadic infections. It seems that the mice become infected at or just after birth and excrete the virus in their urine and droppings for the rest of their lives. Examination of the blood of people living in endemic areas who have never suffered from the illness frequently shows the presence of antibody; hence, mild and subclinical infections must be common.

When Pasteur was working with the rabies virus, he found that when rabbits were inoculated with virus from an infected dog ('street' virus) they took some time to show signs of infection. However, when material from an infected rabbit was passed serially to others, the incubation period of the disease came down to seven days and stayed at that level (now it was called 'fixed' virus). This need for a virus to 'get used to' a new host before causing the quickest and most severe illness seems to be common in nature; people who contract Lassa fever directly from mice usually develop only a mild illness but those who catch it from humans, such as hospital patients, develop a severe illness and frequently die. Thus most of the severe outbreaks of the disease have been centred around hospitals. One further reason for this may be that, in the later stages of fatal cases, the lungs may be full of virus and the act of coughing saturates the environment so that contacts inhale large doses of virus, as is the case in pneumonic plague. (See Chapter 13.)

Between 1969 and 1978 there were 17 outbreaks of the infection in Africa with 386 patients and 105 deaths. Eleven episodes were in hospitals and here the mortality was considerably higher than in other outbreaks.

Ebola fever

Between June and November 1976, an outbreak of infection occurred in the south of the Sudan and the north of Zaire. In Zaire there were 318 cases with 280 deaths, only 38 proved cases surviving. In the Sudan there were 284 cases with 150 deaths. The first case occurred in the Sudan and was a storekeeper in a cotton factory. A second storekeeper became ill but recovered. A third became infected and he, unlike the other two victims, is described as 'an ebullient character'; as well as a bicycle, he had many friends of both sexes, including some who had cared for him in hospital or at home, and he passed on the infection, directly or indirectly, to cause 48 cases and 27 deaths.

When it became obvious that an epidemic was occurring in the region, the Sudanese government put a cordon sanitaire around the area and thus prevented unauthorized persons from moving in or out. An exception was a colleague of mine who was sent by the World Health Organization to investigate. He describes how, when landing at the nearest airstrip, his pilot pushed the landing fee into his hand, hurried him out of the plane and took off again without stopping his engines!

The majority of cases in the Sudan were in those who had cared for infected people either at home or in hospital. The outbreak in Zaire was even more hospital orientated. The local mission hospital had 120 beds and dealt with 6,000 to 12,000 outpatients each month. Five syringes and needles were issued to the nursing staff each morning for use in the hospital, the outpatients' department and the antenatal clinic. These syringes were rinsed in a pan of warm water between uses and were sometimes boiled at the end of the day. About eighty-five cases were probably infected through unsterilized syringes and, as there was an active antenatal clinic, this meant that an unduly large proportion of young women were infected. One hundred and forty-nine persons became infected following contact with patients, usually in their homes in villages, and 43 cases had histories of both contact and injection and so could have been infected either way.

The disease closely resembled that caused by the Marburg virus, together with a resemblance in appearance between the two viruses, but its surface substances (antigens) were quite different. However, it is interesting to note that, when a laboratory worker in Britain became accidentally infected with Ebola virus, he continued to harbour the virus in his semen for weeks after his recovery as did one of the original cases of Marburg virus infection.

The arboviruses

In July 1865 the barque *Hecla* left Cuba and several of her crew of ten became ill during the voyage. When she arrived in Swansea, South Wales about six weeks later, one seaman died soon afterwards although two had recovered. Next to the *Hecla* in Swansea was moored the *Eleanor*; during the following weeks three members of the crew of the

Eleanor and twenty of the other inhabitants of Swansea developed yellow fever and fifteen of the infected persons died. The virus that causes yellow fever is one of the arboviruses; the latter is a large group that affect man and other mammals but which are spread by bites of arthropods (usually mosquitoes, sandflies or ticks) in which they need to develop for some time before they can cause infection. (See Chapter 10.)

The arbovirus group is very widespread but the greatest number of types occurs in Africa. Only about 20 per cent of types cause human infection. After introduction under the skin by the mosquito or other vector, the virus multiplies throughout the body and like other viruses we have discussed different types have different 'target organs', which they damage more so than others. Many of the types found in the USA home in on the brain and cause encephalitis, so that we have Eastern Equine Encephalitis, a disease shared between man and horses; there is also a Western Equine Encephalitis and a St Louis Encephalitis among others.

In 'The Case of the Dying Detective', Sherlock Holmes asked the unfortunate Dr Watson: 'What do you know, pray, of Tapanuli fever? What do you know of the black Formosa corruption?' These names were invented by Conan Doyle (who was a physician) but he could have saved his imagination by looking at a list of arboviruses: Chikungunya, Semliki Forest Fever, O'nyong-nyong, Pixuna, Murray Valley Encephalitis, Kyasanur Forest Disease, Catu, Moju, Simbu, Colorado Tick Fever, Crimean Haemorrhagic Fever, Nakiwogu. These are but a few of the names given to the nearly 500 different types of arbovirus. The very names are, on the whole, so unfamiliar that it seems unlikely that any, apart from yellow fever, are of great importance even in Africa.

When I first drafted this chapter I wrote, 'Yellow fever is at present a rare disease in man'. A few weeks later an article appeared in the medical press which described an outbreak involving several thousand cases with 6,500 deaths in Nigeria! I should not be surprised at anything coming out of Africa. The outbreak was in a remote part where vaccination was either not known or too expensive.

I have talked about the arboviruses at moderate length only to emphasize the vast numbers of different types of virus that exist in Africa and the rest of the Third World – a small change in the constitution of one of these viruses might easily lead to the emergence of an infection rivalling or exceeding AIDS in its seriousness.

Parasitic diseases in the Third World

Although all organisms capable of causing infection or infestation are, strictly speaking, parasites, the word 'parasite' is used particularly for two special categories of infecting agent: the single celled parasites, such as that causing malaria, and the larger worms. These two categories differ from each other in several important ways.

The single celled parasites are of the same *order* of size as bacteria, except that they are slightly larger, so that they are still microscopic; although some embryo worms are very small, the majority of adults may be seen with the naked eye and some are very large, human tape worms reaching thirty feet in length.

In keeping with their small size, the single celled parasites multiply rapidly, as do bacteria; this means that there is ample scope for genetic changes and *the development of resistance to conventional drugs* in the same way that bacteria do. This is best seen in malaria, where resistance to chloroquin – in most cases a safe and reliable drug – has been increasing over the last decade. (In Africa, it is still as easy to contract malaria as it was when Stanley said, 'Doctor Livingstone, I presume', in Ujiji in 1871.) However, as the worms have a much longer life cycle they remain sensitive to drugs that have been used for many years.

Another important difference between these two sorts of parasite is that the single celled parasites are able to multiply within the body – a patient suffering from malaria may have up to 50 per cent of his red blood cells infected. This needs roughly seven million million parasites so that, clearly, a great degree of multiplication must go on within the patient's body. On the other hand the worms almost always need somewhere else for their eggs to develop, either in other animals (snails in the case of the schistosomas) or perhaps only warm soil; in any case multiplication rarely occurs in the body.

This fact has very important consequences; if a single infection of malaria or amoebic dysentery is contracted abroad, the organism can multiply within the patient sufficiently as to cause severe infection or death, even after return to a temperate, parasite-free country. Each year a number of travellers die in Britain as a result of what might be a *single* malarial infection contracted in the tropics. On the other hand, the acquisition of a single worm infection is unlikely to cause severe illness as there will be no increase in the number of parasites within the subject. The whole importance of the worm problem is the risk of constant re-infection so that the most severe conditions occur in those living in an environment where re-infection is frequent. It is here that death occurs and also the chronic illness which has, in the past, been mistaken for laziness and stupidity on the part of the 'native population'.

The following single celled parasites are dealt with:

Malaria
Trypanosomiasis
Leishmaniasis
Amoebic dysentery (See Chapter 9).

Malaria

Malaria is the illness that most people think of when tropical diseases are mentioned. A hundred years or so ago the public was thrilled by news of African exploration and was familiar with the ills and inconveniences of the explorers, particularly those caused by malaria, including the dreaded blackwater fever.

However, malaria is an ancient diseases and was, indeed, common in Britain during the first part of the nineteenth century. Four centuries BC the Greeks were draining marshes to abolish the disease, although they did not know how it was caused. In the second century AD there were several outbreaks of plague in Rome and at the same time malaria gradually spread over that part of Italy. Plague disappeared but malaria remained – as it will if the appropriate mosquitoes remain in the locality. Gradually, over the centuries, the more important marshes in Europe were drained and malaria began to disappear, although it was not until the time of Mussolini that the notorious Pontine Marshes, near Rome, were finally drained.

In Britain malaria was the cause of a fair proportion of cases of 'ague', meaning 'sharp' and describing the onset and course of the disease. For some reason, possibly as a result of the draining of marshes (but this is not very convincing), malaria began to disappear in Britain. In 1840 the main focus here was the Isle of Sheppey, with fewer cases occurring in the Fen Country and in marshy areas bordering the Bristol Channel. In the USA the disease was not eradicated until just before the outbreak of the Second World War.

Where infected subjects are present together with the appropriate mosquitoes, small outbreaks will occur even in areas normally free from the disease; this happened in both Britain and the USA after both world wars and there was a quite sizeable outbreak in Grays, Essex, after the First World War. Cases have also occurred in people living in the vicinity of a Dutch airport but who have never travelled to malarial countries, presumably by mosquitoes that have 'stowed away' on the aircraft when it was in a malarial region.

Chronic malaria, caused by recurring infection in people living in endemic areas, results in tiredness and lethargy and, together with other infestations (particularly those due to worms), accounts to a great extent for the low levels of productivity that occur in the Tropics and for the often unjustified accusations of laziness made by immigrants from a healthier culture against the natives of the warmer countries.

The infection

The disease is caused by a group of small single celled parasites known as plasmodia (single 'plasmodium'). These parasites are acquired through the bite of an infected female mosquito and their life cycle falls into three parts:

1. *In the patient's liver.* The malarial parasite is present in the mosquito's saliva which is used by the insect to prevent clotting of the blood it removes from the patient. From the saliva the organisms get into the wound, then into the small blood vessels and, by way of the blood, to the liver. Here they enter liver cells and multiply within them. They continue to multiply for one or two weeks and then burst back into the blood. Fortunately, in the most severe form of malaria, none of the parasites remain dormant in the liver, but other types of malarial parasites are liable to, so that repeated recurrence of infection can happen over long periods. Malaria may be contracted by transfusion of infected blood; however, in this case the parasites never enter the liver but enter red cells directly. Thus, whatever the type of malaria contracted by blood transfusion, recurrence does not take place. (See Figure 11.1.)

2. *In the patient's blood.* Once they pass from the liver to the blood, the parasites, now in large numbers, enter red cells – usually only one per cell, although the type of parasite that causes severe malaria may have several parasites per cell. Within the red cell, the parasites once again begin to multiply until they fill the cell; the latter now ruptures and releases the parasites and their presence, unprotected by the red cell, causes fever and shivering; because many parasites will have entered their red cells at the same time and, as they multiply at approximately the same rate, they are all likely to rupture the cells at the same time. Because they take either forty-eight or seventy-two hours to mature depending on the type of malarial parasite infecting, at the onset fevers occur either every second or third day, when all the infected red cells

Figure 11.1 Malaria cycle in patient's liver

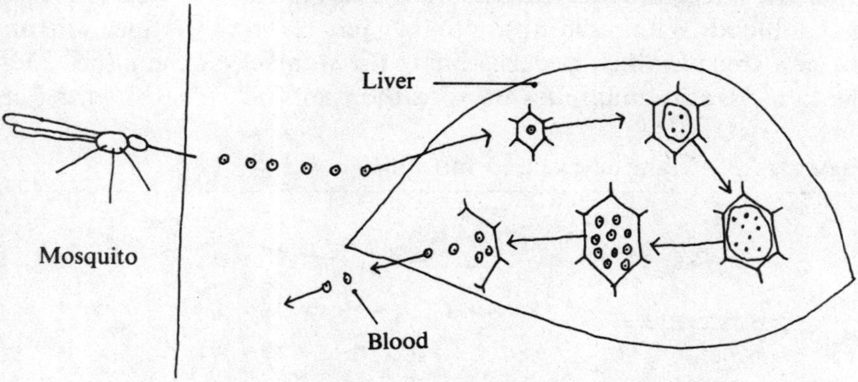

The parasites enter the blood following a mosquito bite and pass to the liver. They multiply within the liver cells for several days and then burst back into the blood.

burst at the same time. Later in the illness the parasites begin to rupture red cells 'out of phase' so that the fever becomes continuous. Up until now, all the offspring of the original parasites will have been roughly spherical but, at a certain stage of the infection, there appear a few sexual forms (gametes) which are sausage shaped. They indulge in no sexual activity in the patient but do so in the next stage. (See Figure 11.2.)

Figure 11.2 Malarial cycle in patient's blood

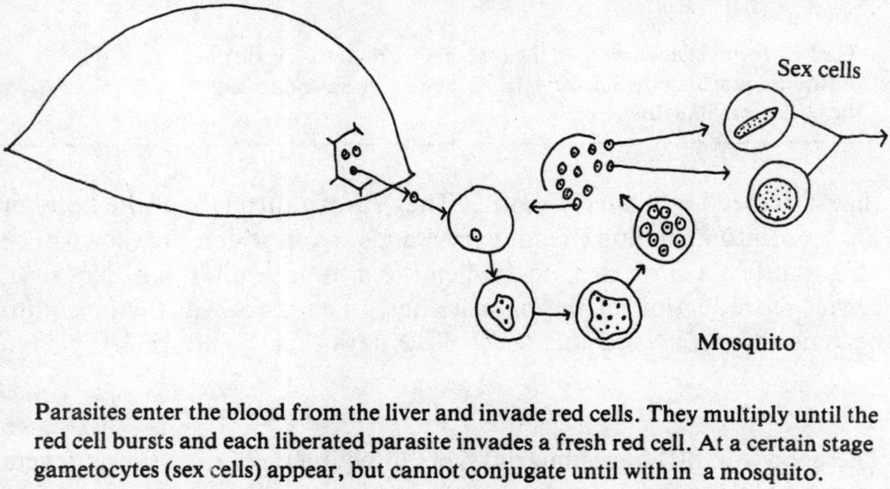

Parasites enter the blood from the liver and invade red cells. They multiply until the red cell bursts and each liberated parasite invades a fresh red cell. At a certain stage gametocytes (sex cells) appear, but cannot conjugate until with in a mosquito.

3. *In the mosquito.* When an uninfected mosquito draws blood from the infected patient, a few male and female cells will be present in that blood. Within the mosquito they join together (fertilization) and the new organism invades cells lining the stomach of the insect. Here the new parasite multiplies up to a thousandfold. The offspring are

Figure 11.3 Malarial cycle in mosquito

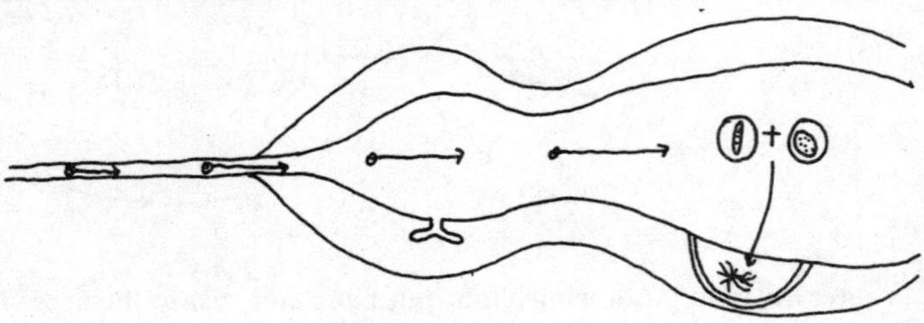

The mosquito bites, withdrawing blood that contains malarial sex cells. These conjugate and multiply within a cyst in the mosquito's stomach wall.

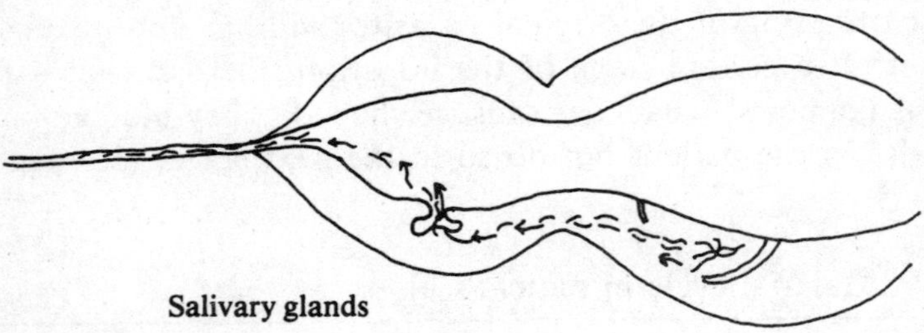

The tiny forms that develop in the cyst on the stomach invade the body of the mosquito, reaching the salivary glands. When the mosquito bites again it transmits the parasite in its saliva.

threadshaped and actively motile. They spread throughout the body of the mosquito including the salivary glands, from which site they will be able to infect a further patient when the mosquito bites him. Not until sexual reproduction of the parasite has taken place will the mosquito become infectious and this takes 8–12 days (See Figure 11.3.)

Different types of malarial parasites

There are four different malarial types infecting humans, although there are many others that infect mammals and birds. The human types differ slightly in appearance when seen under the microscope but more so in the rate at which they multiply, the severity of the disease they cause and the likelihood of the infection relapsing. The four types are called *Plasmodium falciparum*, *Pl. malariae*, *Pl. vivax* and *Pl. ovale*.

Pl. falciparum is the most important one for visitors to the Tropics because it can cause a fatal illness. All patients who die from malaria on return to Britain from a trip abroad die from *Pl. falciparum* infection. The disease caused by this parasite is known as 'malignant tertian' malaria – 'malignant' because of the severe infection caused and 'tertian' (third) because, at least during the first week or so the illness, the patient suffers attacks of fever on the first and third days; the name is not very logical as, in fact, fever occurs every *second* day. Because latent forms of this type do not persist in the liver, relapses do not occur after the original illness. However, the organism, unlike the other types of malarial parasite, can develop in red cells of all ages and parasitize up to 50 per cent of the cells and for this reason infections are serious.

Pl. vivax and *Pl. ovale* can only parasitize young red cells so that they cannot destroy as many as *Pl. falciparum* can; hence, single infections are rarely fatal. However, latent forms can persist in the liver, causing recurrences for up to forty years, in Westerners often long after their return from the Tropics. *Pl. vivax* and *Pl. ovale*, like *Pl. falciparum*, take about forty-eight hours to mature in a red cell so that they cause 'benign tertian' malaria.

Pl. malariae resembles *Pl. vivax* and *Pl. ovale* in relative mildness and liability to recurrence but, as it takes seventy-two hours to mature in red cells, it produces fever every *third* day, causing 'benign quartan' malaria.

The problem of malaria

Although malaria has been eliminated from most of Europe, it is still a cause of many deaths and much illness throughout the world. Estimates of its prevalence differ; it has been said that, at any one time, there are 10 million cases in the world with one million deaths annually; another estimate is that there are one million deaths each year in Africa alone.

In 1955 the World Health Organization began a drive to eradicate malaria completely. By 1976 this programme was officially declared a failure. The failure was due mainly to the development of resistance to the antimalarial drugs in use. As we saw earlier, the rapid multiplication rate of the malarial parasite allows for large numbers of mutations, some of which help the organism to avoid the lethal effects of the drugs used.

In Britain blood transfusion or the sharing of syringes by drug addicts is a very rare cause of infection but in the USA it is not uncommon; fortunately the disease, when contracted in this way, does not recur.

Avoiding and treating malaria

It is generally believed that malaria did not reach the Americas until after discovery by Columbus so that it would seem possible that malaria might have been a fair exchange for syphilis. However, the Amazonian Indians discovered that malaria could be cured with 'cinchona', obtained from the bark of a local tree. The drug was brought to England in 1632 as a secret remedy, by the Jesuits. It gained its name from the Countess of Chinchon, the wife of the Spanish Viceroy (she is sometimes referred to, inaccurately, as the 'vice queen'!). After its introduction it was used indiscriminately in treating all fevers but the only condition it cured was malaria; it is still used in tonics and also to improve the flavour of gin! Louis XIV of France contracted malaria and was cured by quinine. Oliver Cromwell and possibly King James I also developed malaria and perhaps died from it.

During the Second World War supplies of quinine were limited and other drugs were developed, notably mepacrine and then chloroquin. Although the latter is still the drug of choice for the prevention of malaria in most parts, more and more areas are acquiring malarial parasites resistant to it so that visitors to the Tropics should acquire expert advice upon what prophylactic drug to take according to the location they intend to visit. In Britain this can be easily obtained by telephoning the Malaria Reference Laboratory at the London School of Hygiene.

As antimalarial drugs affect mainly the parasite in the blood and not that in the liver, it is important to continue taking the drug for 6 weeks after return from a malarious area; it is also recommended that the drug be taken for at least 1 week before commencing the visit.

Prophylactic drugs are not the only means of preventing malaria; simple precautions such as keeping the arms and legs covered after sundown, the use of mosquito nets and of insect repellants and the avoidance of marsh areas all play an important part in preventing infection. I noted with sadness the obituary to my former commanding officer in Egypt, who regarded catching malaria as a self-inflicted injury. When he became ill, I, as pathologist, had to examine his blood films over a long period before I found a malarial parasite—but I succeeded in the end!

Sickle cell anaemia

This interesting hereditary condition affects mainly Meditarranean and black people. The haemoglobin in the red cells of these patients has a slightly different chemical constitution from the normal. As a result cells tend to break down spontaneously during attacks called 'crises' (often precipitated by a virus infection) so that the patients suffer from severe anaemia. However, the red cells of these patients are more resistant to malaria than normal red cells. It seems that, in the countries where this abnormality arose, resistance to malaria was an advantage that outweighed the disadvantage of possible anaemia so that those who possessed this abnormal haemoglobin survived and multiplied better than those without it.

Trypanosomiasis

In the sixteenth and seventeenth centuries the Portuguese sent several expeditions to Africa, especially along the Zambesi, in search of gold mines. These expeditions depended upon horses for transport but these animals died one by one as a result of bites from a fly now known as the tsetse fly; the members of the expedition were then destroyed in equal measure by local diseases and the local population. The disease carried by the flies is known as 'nagana' and is caused by a small single celled parasite.

In 1843 a French scientist was looking at frog's blood under the microscope and saw a small organism that moved with a spiral motion so he called it a 'trypanosome', literally a 'boring body'. The disease nagana is caused by trypanosomes as are several other diseases in animals and man. If it had not been for this organism, the Portuguese might well have conquered most of Africa and the course of history in Africa might have been very different.

The organism

Although there are minor differences, all trypanosomes are very similar, being torpedo shaped with a nucleus, a membrane and a tail. Three species are important to man, the Gambian strain and the Rhodesian strain in Africa and *Trypanosoma cruzi* in South America.

Trypanosome infections in humans

In Africa the trypanosomes cause sleeping sickness and related conditions. In West and Central Africa the Gambian strain is spread by the tsetse fly and its relatives. The only source is man, so that there is a 'man - fly - man' cycle. About 10,000 new cases occur each year. Once signs of the disease appear death is inevitable in a year unless treatment is given. The patient suffers from psychosis, hallucinations, mania or depressions. He gradually becomes more comatose, then emaciated and subsequently dies.

In East Africa the Rhodesian strain has more or less the same effect; however, the parasite infects antelopes and other game animals as well as domestic cattle so that man may be infected by flies feeding on these animals. About 1,500 cases are reported in East Africa each year but the real number infected must be many times as great.

In South America there are some unpleasant bugs that inhabit the houses. These are over an inch in length and they feed at night on the blood of man and domestic animals, resembling, in some ways, bed bugs. Even their feeding habits are unpleasant because they regularly defaecate on the skin of the patient. Their faeces contain *T. cruzi*, which the patient may scratch into the wound made by the bug with its blood-sucking apparatus or may contaminate his hands and hence his nose or lips. Millions of infections occur, there being approximately ten million infected persons in Brazil alone. The infection may continue for twenty years and is particularly likely to be fatal in young children. There is no really suitable drug available for treatment. The organism attacks particularly the brain and the heart—it has been said that if a mad South American drops dead from heart failure he must have been a victim of Chagas' disease.

South American trypanosomiasis

This condition is a classic example of a disease which affects millions and kills thousands each year that could be wiped out completely by a single substance—money! If the walls of the dwellings inhabited by millions of South Americans were brought up to the standard of those in houses inhabited by even the poorest people in Britain, the reduviid bugs—and the vast majority of cases of Chagas' disease—would disappear, just as the bed bug has practically disappeared from Britain.

While the trypanosomes are the cause of millions of infections and deaths throughout the world, the infection is practically unknown in Britain. Charles Darwin, who developed the theory of evolution, spent five years in or near South America between 1831 and 1836. on his return he became a chronic invalid; he eventually had a heart attack in 1873 and died from another in 1882. His illness, particularly the intestinal and heart symptoms, resembles Chagas' disease and he was, indeed, badly bitten by one of the reduviid bugs in 1835, so that the diagnosis is not unlikely.

Leishmaniasis

The African trypanosomes do not penetrate the cells of the body but the South American variety do. They penetrate and multiply in, many types of tissue cell. However, once inside the cell, they lose their flagellum and undulating membrane, becoming somewhat featureless oval bodies with two nuclei. This is of great interest to those who are interested in tracing the development of different forms of parasite, because the group we are now discussing, the leishmania, look exactly like the South American trypanosomes when they are located within cells. These

Figure 11.4 Different forms of the trypanosome family

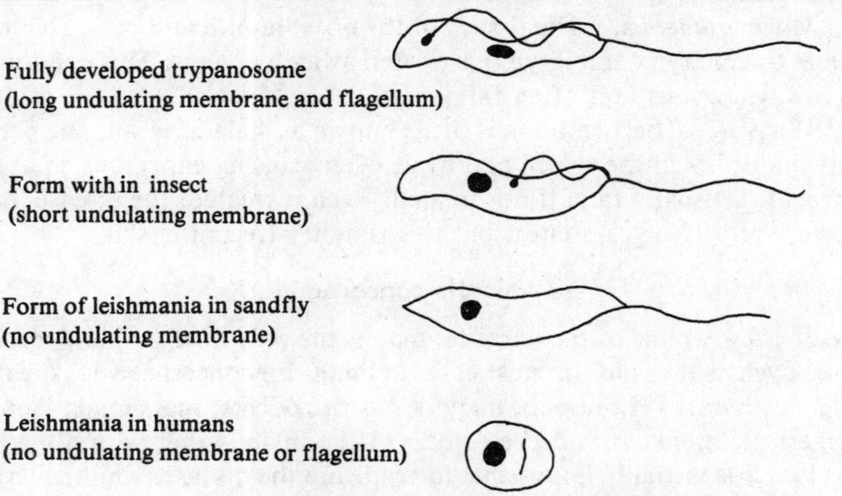

parasites are carried by sandflies and within the insect they develop a short flagellum so that they roughly resemble certain forms of the African trypanosomes; there is little doubt that these two groups are closely related. (See Figure 11.4.)

Life cycle

The infection is transmitted by sandflies. The parasites need to develop at least ten days within this insect before they can be successfully transmitted. They develop into the form with the flagellum and multiply so actively that they produce a partial blockage of the sandfly's foregut and, in an attempt to clear the blockage, the sandfly forcibly expels the parasites with its saliva.

Entering the human host through the sandfly's proboscis, the parasites, now having lost their flagella, are ingested by those white cells whose duty it is to destroy foreign bodies. However, the leishmania are not destroyed by being swallowed in this way; indeed, they are protected from noxious outside influences, such as antibody, and they multiply unconcernedly within the cell. When that cell dies the parasites are released and then ingested by further white cells and thus the infection progresses.

From now on the development of the disease varies according to the strain of parasite causing the infection. There are three types of disease:

1. *Cutaneous.* Ulcers form on the skin and usually clear up without treatment.
2. *Mucocutaneous.* The tissues of the nose, mouth and palate (sometimes the pharynx and larynx) are eaten away by ulcers. This condition is always serious and often fatal.
3. *Visceral.* This condition is often known as 'kala-azar' and the parasite multiplies in the spleen and liver, often causing enormous enlargement. It is usually fatal if not treated. Even if treated, the disease may recur up to five years later, but this time it affects the skin.

Animals concerned

With a few strains of the parasite, man is the only host so that a man – man cycle is the rule. In most cases animals are concerned: dogs, cats, jackals, hyraxes (Ethiopia), many kinds of rodents, marsupials (South America), monkeys and even sloths. It is obvious that with all these vectors it is virtually impossible to eradicate the disease from the environment. Treatment is by injection of antimony compounds; although many cases of cutaneous leishmaniasis will heal when treated with local antiseptics or antibiotics as necessary, the other types need vigorous treatment to save life.

The problem of leishmaniasis

There is a scenario known as the 'pink toothbrush' situation which arises through reading with only half an eye or listening with only half an ear. The name arose like this:

Many years ago, in the USA, there was a radio programme on dental hygiene which stressed the importance of bleeding from the gums as a warning signal; this was indicated by the slightly bloodstained bristles of the toothbrush – hence 'pink toothbrush'. For some time after the broadcast drug stores were inundated by customers who had jettisoned their old blue-, red- or green-handled toothbrush and were anxious to buy the 'recommended' pink toothbrush!

The same principle inspires the concern felt by two friends of mine. Some weeks earlier there had been published in a national newspaper an article on leishmaniasis that appeared to be intended to inflate the writer's ego rather than inform the public. On the basis of a series of one case of the disease being contracted by a British holidaymaker, leishmaniasis was pictured as a menacing disease slowly but inexorably moving towards Britain and liable, eventually, to destroy Western civilization. The disease was stated to resemble malaria, influenza and AIDS. Those who have read this book up to this point will be aware that that these diseases have very little in common so that it would seem impossible for a fourth disease to resemble them all. The writer described how the disease is spread by the sandfly.

Some weeks later my friend explained how he had killed 'a couple of those insects that spread AIDS – there was an article in the paper about it!' I understood, on recalling the article, that he meant sandflies. 'One bit my wife,' he went on, 'so we rang up the writer of the article but he didn't seem very interested.' How did the sandflies arrive in the rain-forests of darkest Essex in late November, I wondered. There was an easy answer to that – they were carried over by the wind that occasionally brings sand-laden rain from the Sahara.

Despite the above, leishmaniasis is not likely to cause any significant infection in Britain, although it is only prudent for travellers abroad to take steps to avoid insect bites and to treat any that occur with a suitable disinfectant cream or lotion.

TWELVE

A Trip to the Tropics II

Of all the organisms that inflict man, the worms are without doubt the most fascinating. The unqualified word 'worm' today indicates, usually, the common earthworm but, in earlier times, a more fearsome beast was indicated. Just before his last battle King Arthur dreamed that he sat on a chair which was fast to a wheel and there was under 'him an hideous black water, and therein were all manner of serpents, and worms and wild beasts, foul and horrible; and suddenly the king thought the wheel turned up-so-down and he fell among the serpents and every beast took him by a limb'. Conversely, there has been a suggestion that the Guinea worm (*Dracunculus medinensis*) was the 'fiery serpent' inflicted upon the Children of Israel.

One of the attractions of the worms is the large size of some of them—the infecting agent may often be seen and appreciated by the layman without the help of a microscope or other laboratory equipment. The Guinea worm may measure two to four feet in length; the fish tapeworm may exceed thirty-three feet in length and in the seventeenth century, Tyson, recorded that a patient passed 800 feet of tapeworm in a year.

At the other extreme are the minute microfilaria, larval forms of larger worms, that may be present in the blood and which must be sought with a microscope. Between these extremes there are a large number of organisms varying in length from considerably less than an inch to a few inches.

Another fascinating aspect of the study of worms is the convoluted lifestyle adopted by many of them, some of which need as many as three or more hosts in order to fulfil their life span completely. The host in which the adult worm resides is regarded as the 'definitive' host and the others are 'intermediate'; however, some of the worms perform a variation on their usual theme in that man may be both the definitive and the intermediate host. This may seem difficult to understand but will be explained at greater length later.

The following worms are considered here (it should be noted that this is not a scientific classification):

1. Worms introduced through the mouth – by contaminated hands, etc.
   Ascaris lumbricoides
   Enterobius vermicularis (the threadworm, pinworm or seat-worm)
   Dracunculus medinensis (the Guinea worm)
2. Worms introduced through the mouth – by contaminated food (usually meat)
   Tapeworms
   Trichinella spiralis (the Little Spiral Hair)
3. Worms introduced through the skin – directly
   Hookworms
   Schistosomes
4. Worms introduced through the skin – by insects
   Filaria (including *Onchocerca volvulus* – river blindness)

Worms introduced through the mouth
By contaminated hands, etc.

Ascaris lumbricoides

One of the commonest of parasitic worms, it has affected man at least since the stone age. It is a relatively large worm, measuring up to twelve inches in length and usually about one sixth of an inch in width. 'Lumbricoides' means 'resembling the earthworm' and there is some resemblance. Eggs of this worm are moderately resistant and can frequently pass through sewage treatment plants without being killed.

In a town in Germany where more than half of the inhabitants were suffering from ascaris infection, the sewage was treated and the effluent passed to a village outside the town. Here it was used to irrigate salad plants, which were then passed back to the town and eaten raw. Eggs of ascaris were present on the salad material and, thus, the citizens of that German town got their own back and with interest. The villagers also ate their salads untreated and developed an even higher level of ascaris infection.

Life cycle

Once eaten by man (this worm does not infect other animals) the eggs, which can exist in damp earth for at least five years, release the small larvae which bore their way through the wall of the small bowel and enter the blood stream. They arrive at the liver where they pause for a while. They then pass back to the blood and move with it to the heart, from which they are transported to the lungs. Here most of them break out of the air sacs (alveoli) into the air passages; from here they are wafted upwards, coughed up and then swallowed to reach the bowel again. They pass to the small bowel from whence their odessey started, mature and begin to lay eggs. Quite often a few larvae remain in the lung, where they mature, and it is said that there are few people in the West Indies who have not coughed up a mature ascaris at some time or other. (See Figure 12.1.)

Figure 12.1 *Ascaris lumbricoides* life cycle

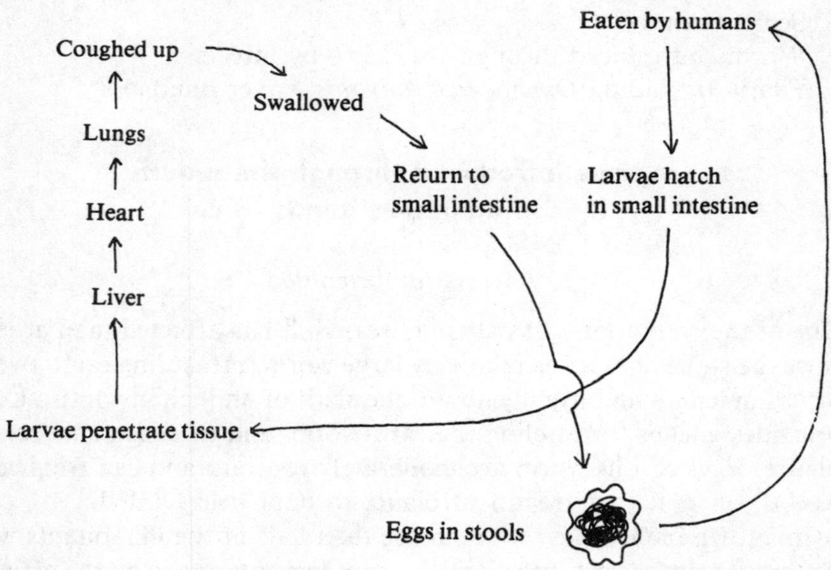

Prevalence

Although rare in Britain, this condition occurs in most other parts of the world and, in 1947, it was estimated that 644 million people in the world harboured this worm. In China alone, some 335 million people were believed to be infected and it was calculated that 18,000 tons of eggs were produced annually!

The illness

If only a few worms are present, their effect is slight but larger numbers can cause indigestion, abdominal pain, diarrhoea and enteritis. Worms in the liver and in the appendix can cause jaundice and appendicitis, respectively. They affect rarely the ear or the genito-urinary system.

Avoidance

Avoidance costs money and involves the introduction of sewage treatment systems that kill the eggs of the worm. Refraining from eating fresh salads and uncooked fruits (the disease can be contracted from strawberries) and the thorough washing of such uncooked food that has to be eaten help to prevent infection.

Enterobius vermicularis

This worm is usually known as the threadworm but is also known as the pinworm or seat-worm (for obvious reasons). It is the only worm common in Britain but here, as elsewhere, it may be found in all social strata, not excluding the seats of the mighty. It is a small worm, the larger female not exceeding half an inch in length.

Life cycle

The worms live within the intestine in the region of the appendix (and they have been suspected of causing appendicitis). Once the female has been fertilized she begins her journey down the intestine and, usually in the night, passes out through the anus. Here conditions are too much for her and she literally explodes, scattering her eggs around the region of the bottom. The movement of the female in the area of the anus causes the itching, which is about the only symptom of infection (occasionally the worms may colonize the vagina, causing more itching and greater embarrassment).

Three things may happen to the eggs laid around the posterior:

1. *Autoinfection*. The subject scratches his bottom and then puts his hand to his mouth. Although the lifespan of this worm is only a few weeks, infection can last indefinitely as a result of this autoinfection. It is commonly described as 'Parasites lost—Parasites regained'.

2. *Retrofection.* Some of the eggs in the perianal region may hatch and the larvae crawl back through the anus, keeping the infection going indefinitely.
3. *Crossinfection.* The eggs are present in the underclothes and also on the bedding. They are spread throughout the environment by bed-making and other active manipulations of infected garments. In an infected household the eggs may be found with ease in the house dust.

(See Figure 12.2.)

Figure 12.2 Threadworms

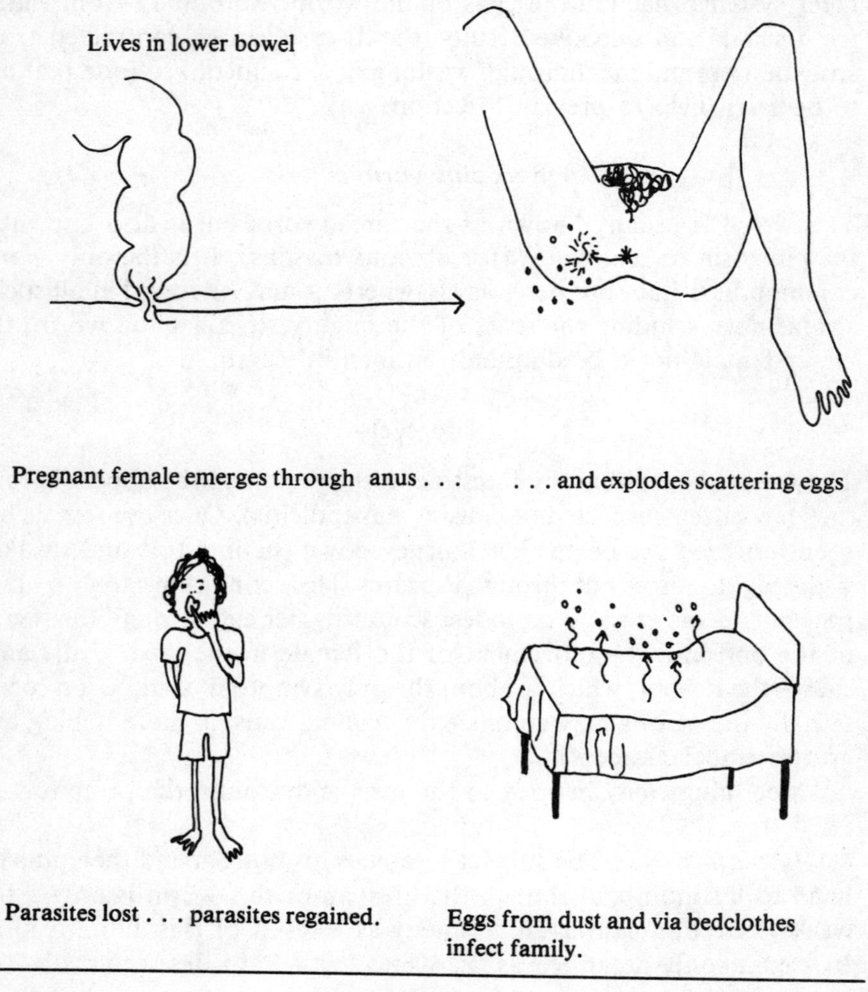

Diagnosis and avoidance

Diagnosis may be made from the symptoms and the occasional presence of female worms in the stools. To be quite certain, it is only necessary to apply the sticky side of a piece of cellulose tape to the region around the anus and then to put the sticky side on to a microscope slide. Under the microscope the eggs have a typical appearance, being oval with one side flattened.

Although these worms do little physical harm, adults harbouring them suffer severe psychological effects, usually in the form of a guilt complex, akin to the feelings of those whose hair harbours headlice. For this reason alone, treatment is recommended and there are some efficient drugs. However, some extra considerations are necessary; all members of the family must be treated at the same time, the treatment must be repeated fourteen days later and special attention must be paid to the washing of underclothes and bedlinen and to 'spring-cleaning' in order to remove dust that might be infectious.

Dracunculus medinensis

'And the Lord sent fiery serpents among the people and they bit the people: and much people of Israel died.' This passage from the Book of Numbers probably describes an outbreak of Guinea worm infection among the Children of Israel. At that time they were in the vicinity of the Gulf of Akaba, where this infection is widespread. About 300 miles away is the second most holy Moslem city, Medina, and the disease must have occurred there frequently to have earned its name. At the worm is very long and very thin, it was thought, in the Middle Ages, to have been a vein that had undergone degenerative changes and it was called Vena Medina—the Medina vein. When it was shown, later to be a worm, it became *Dracunculus medinensis*—the Little Dragon of Medina. It is usually known as the Guinea worm.

The worm and its life cycle

This worm is found in Africa (the Nile Valley and central and equatorial Africa) and in the Middle East and India. The female worm measures from two to four feet in length but less than a tenth of an inch in diameter. The male is only about half an inch in length and is rarely seen. As well as man, they can infect dogs, wolves, baboons, hares and other animals.

The female lives in the tissues for ten to fourteen months, at first producing no symptoms, but all this time she has been producing, in her womb, millions of active larvae, so many that her food canal disappears to make room for the offspring. She now has to discharge her larvae into the outside world, which is done by her migrating to a part of the body that is likely to be immersed in cold water, such as the arms, chest, abdomen or lower limbs.

When the worm's head reaches the skin, a blister appears which may reach two inches in diameter. If cold water is poured over this blister, an ulcer is formed and a milky fluid consisting of thousands of small larvae appears. This is the natural way that the larvae escape to the environment. Once in water, the larvae swim about; most of them die but a few may be eaten by a small water-flea (Cyclops). Within the water-flea the larvae bore their way from the food canal to the blood space, where they develop into infectious larvae. It now only remains for water containing infected water-fleas to be drunk by a human and the cycle of infection recommences. The digestive enzymes in the stomach digest the water-flea and release the larvae, which bore their way out of the stomach and reach the distant tissues where they develop into adult males and females.

Treatment and avoidance

The traditional method is to roll the worm up on a stick, extracting only a few centimetres a day so as not to break the worm. This process is made easier by treating the patient with a drug that kills the worm, such as metranidazole. In other cases, the worm may be removed under local anaesthesia after its position has been determined by X-rays.

Prevention is by boiling water used for drinking and, on a larger scale, chlorination or treatment of domestic water supplies with copper sulphate.

Worms introduced through the mouth
By contaminated food

Tapeworms and their relatives

The Israelites were forbidden to eat pork, as are Moslems who appeared later but in roughly the same part of the world. This was almost certainly in order to reduce the risk of contracting the pork tapeworm, *Taenia solium*, but, unfortunately, this purely public health precept has been petrified into a religious precept long after the health need for it has disappeared.

Tapeworms must have been common in Britain in the past, because there is still a lively folk belief that any thin person with a ravenous appetite must be 'suffering from worms'. Today, the pork tapeworm is no longer found in Britain and even the beef tapeworm. *Taenia saginata*, is rare.

Life cycles

Tapeworms have two phases of existence: in their definitive host they take the form of a worm, while in the intermediate host they exist as a bladder-like cyst. (See Figure 12.3.) The arrangement is very simple: the intermediate host eats food contaminated by eggs from the tapeworm. The eggs hatch within this host and the larvae find their way to the muscles, etc. Here they become small cysts that can develop no further in that host. The intermediate host is eaten by the definitive host,

Figure 12.3 The beef tapeworm

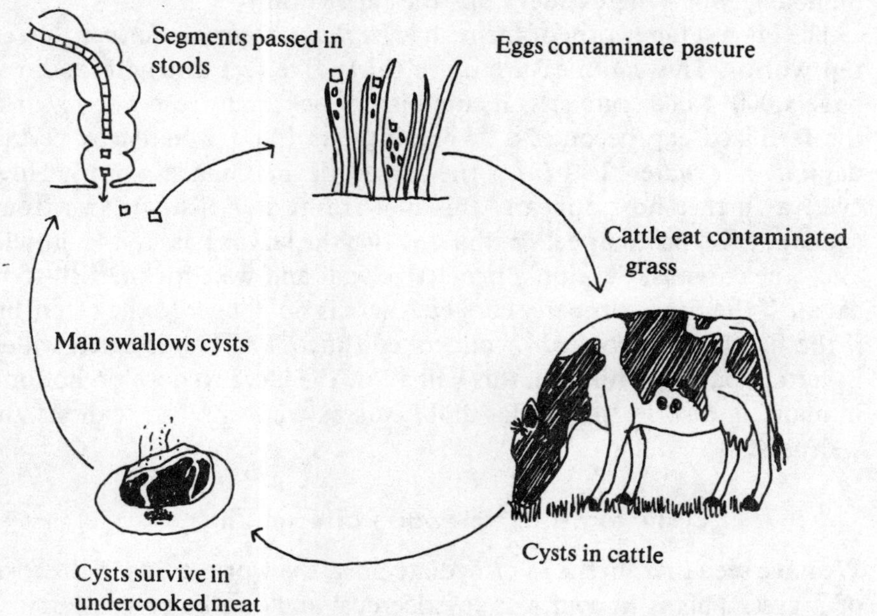

its flesh is digested and the cyst, which contains the head of the worm 'inside-out', inflates the head, like the toy that consists of a ball containing a little man (squeeze the ball and the little man is blown up and stands erect over the hole he emerged from). The head of the worm now attaches itself to the small bowel with suckers or hooks (or both) and proceeds to produce segments. These eventually come to resemble a roll of bus tickets, except that they differ in size as the worm is passed down.

The upper ones are immature; lower down the male reproductive organs begin to appear; then the female organs; eggs are fertilized and the lowest segments consist simply of bags of fertilized eggs.

The segments at the bottom of the chain become detached, those of the beef tapeworm singly and those of the pork tapeworm in groups. These pass out with the faeces and, if they fall on to a suitable area, may be eaten by cattle and the cycle is repeated. The pork tapeworm ova develop in pigs, but this worm occurs mainly in Africa.

Other tapeworms

The hosts used by tapeworms have to be associated in some way or the worm would never survive. For instance, there is a cat/mouse tapeworm; the mouse eats food contaminated by cat droppings and the cysts develop within it; the mouse is eaten by the cat and gets its revenge posthumously when the cat develops the tapeworm.

The biggest tapeworm of them all is *Diphyllobothrium latum* (the fish tapeworm). This can measure up to thirty-five feet in length and may have 3,000–4,000 segments. Its life history begins in fresh water, where the fertilized egg becomes a swimming larva and is eaten by certain daphnia-like water-fleas (as is the case with the Guinea worm). However, a further host appears; this is a freshwater fish such as trout, salmon, pike, perch or eel. Within the fish the larvae pass to the muscles and other organs, develop a protective wall and wait for the fish to be eaten. If the fish is properly cooked, there is no danger to the eater; but if the fish is undercooked or uncooked (uncooked fish is eaten widely in certain parts of Europe), this will allow the larva to develop not only in man but also in foxes, pigs and bears as well as seals, sealions and walruses.

Cystic forms of tapeworm affecting humans

We have seen that, in the intermediate host, the worm exists in the form of a cyst. This is known as a 'cysticercus' and can be seen as a small spherical object in 'measly' pork or beef. An experienced meat inspector can recognize one with ease. If man swallows food contaminated by the ova of the pork tapeworm (and these can only have come from another human) then he acts as the 'intermediate' host and cysticerci develop in his body. These may occur in the heart muscle or brain, causing, at times, severe symptoms.

Another condition in which man occurs as the intermediate host is that of hydatid cyst. This is the cystic form of a worm called *Echinococcus granulosis* which shares most of its life between dogs and sheep (another significant partnership). Within the dog it takes the form of a tiny tapeworm and in the sheep its cystic form resembles the cysticercus of beef. People working closely with dogs and sheep tend to become infected, the eggs in the dog's faeces contaminating its coat, so that, after stroking or patting the dog, the owner may convey some eggs to his mouth. The larva that develops from the egg penetrates the wall of the intestine and passes via the blood to various organs, especially the liver and the lungs. Here it develops into a cyst that is about half an inch in size after five months. If this cyst should develop in the eye or brain or in the 'pacemaking' region of the heart, its effects could be serious, causing fits or heart failure. In the liver it may become extremely large and the cyst contains smaller daughter and even granddaughter cysts inside the daughter cysts. These are infectious so that, if the cyst is to be removed by surgery, it is of greatest importance that no spillage should take place into the body or further cysts will arise at the site of the operation. (See Figure 12.4.)

In 1868 the Earl of Shaftesbury developed a cyst just below his ribs. It was opened and the description of its appearance makes it likely that it was a hydatid cyst. Although all the fluid was removed, it continued to discharge and the surgeons decided to leave a silver drainage tube with a tap in place so that accumulating fluid could be drawn off as necessary. Whether the treatment worked we do not know but Shaftesbury lived on until 1683.

Avoiding tapeworms and their cysts

The three tapeworms most important to man can be avoided by not eating raw meat. Freezing is also lethal to the cysts so that a week or so in a domestic deep freeze will destroy the activity of any cysts present. The worms may be attacked at other points in their development—treatment of drinking water to destroy the water flea will also destroy the larvae of the fish tapeworm. It is known that tapeworm ova may pass through many sewage treatment systems without being killed, although the newer types of plant *do* kill at least 90 per cent of eggs. However, the expense of updating sewage treatment works simply to reduce tapeworm eggs is not justified. Tapeworms occur less and less frequently in Britain and North America chiefly because of the prevalence of refrigerators, the freezing of most meat and the reticence on the part of the consumer to eating uncooked meat. Steak tartare is an

Figure 12.4 Hydatid cyst

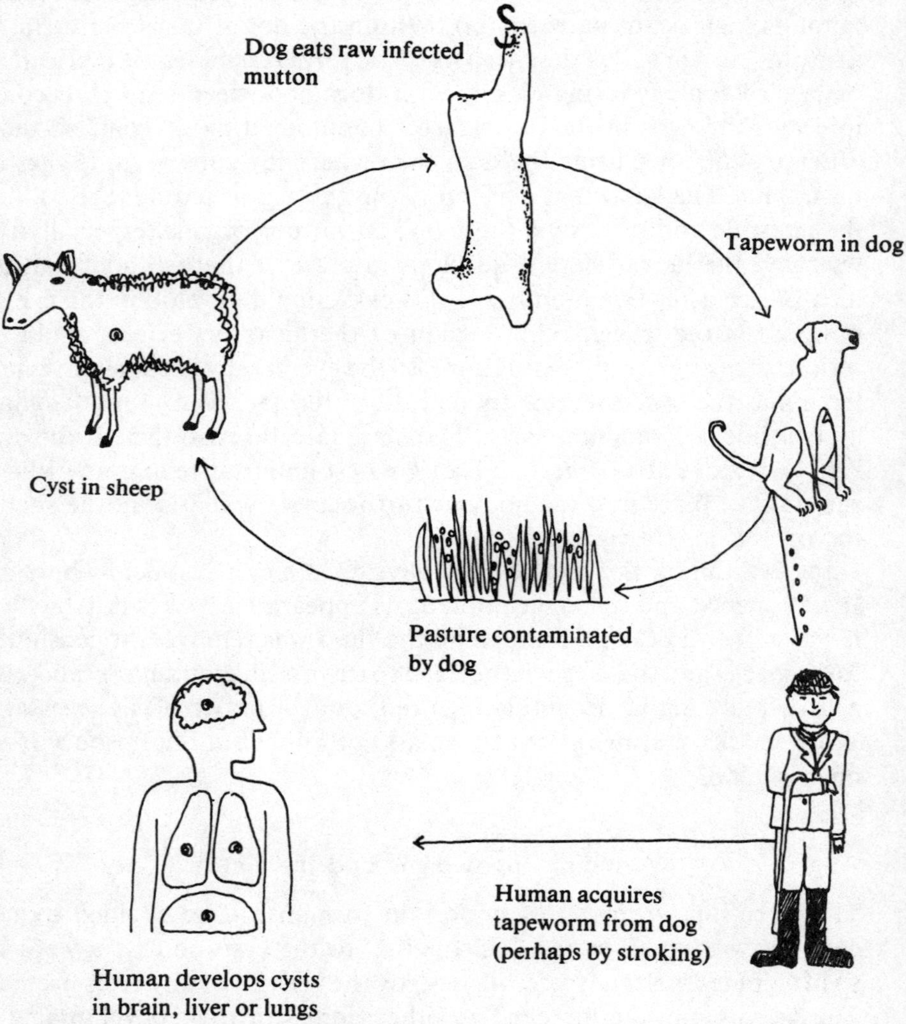

exception to the last statement and should be avoided on principle.

Hydatid cysts occur mainly in areas where dogs and sheep are close to man: Australia, New Zealand, parts of Wales and, formerly, Iceland. In the last country, the cyst was common in the nineteenth century, and about one in four inhabitants was infected. Legislation was introduced to reduce this incidence. Dogs were taxed in an attempt to reduce their total numbers, carcasses with cysts had to be burned and it was forbidden to feed dogs on raw offal. Dogs also had to be wormed annually. It was also emphasized that dogs and man should not come into intimate contact. These measures have resulted in the disappearance of new cases of hydatid cyst in Iceland, the cysts being found post-mortem in only those born before the changes in behaviour.

Trichinella spiralis

Here, for a change, we have a worm that is more prevalent in the Arctic than in the Tropics. *Trichinella spiralis* (the little spiral hair) is a tiny worm, less than one eighth of an inch in length, and, after infection has been established, the female gives birth to larvae in the small bowel of the host. These are carried by the blood to muscles all over the body, where they form tiny cysts that become 'gritty' as they become covered with calcium carbonate. The cysts now wait hopefully for the piece of muscle in which they are residing to be eaten by another host. This rarely occurs naturally in man so that the life cycle of the worm comes to an end. However, if the infection is in a pig which is killed for meat and the remains are fed to healthy pigs, the latter will become infected and the infection is kept alive. The worm is not particular about its choice of host: man, domestic and wild pigs, brown and polar bears, seals and walruses and many game animals may be infected. (See Figure 12.5.)

The illness

Illness is caused by the migration of the larvae in the body and their presence in the muscles. Diagnosis is best made by cutting out a small fragment of muscle and looking for the cysts. The number of cysts per gram of muscle can be determined and this affects the outcome of the illness. Most infections are mild with less than 10 cysts per gram. When there are about 100 cysts per gram, then a typhoid-like illness occurs. Cases with over 2000 cysts per gram are almost always fatal, death occurring after about 6 weeks of illness. Fortunately most cases are mild today. However, in 1865 there was an outbreak in a small town in Germany; 337 of the 2,000 inhabitants were infected and 101 died. The disease is commoner in countries where raw pork is eaten, e.g. Russia, Poland and Germany. The introduction of home freezers and the practice of freezing meat has, as in the case of tapeworm infestation, no doubt played a large part in the near disappearance of this infection as the larvae are killed quite quickly by freezing. Cooking, too, kills the larvae rapidly but, when dealing with a large joint of pork, it is sometimes difficult to ensure that the interior reaches the desired temperature of over 65°C. A practical test is that, if the juices coming out of the joint are still pink, the meat needs further cooking. It is said that the taking of a drink of Irish whiskey with the pork reduces the risk of infection but it is not known if lesser makes of spirit have the same effect!

At present the main sufferers are the Eskimo people, of whom about 59 per cent are said to be affected.

Figure 12.5 Trichinella spiralis

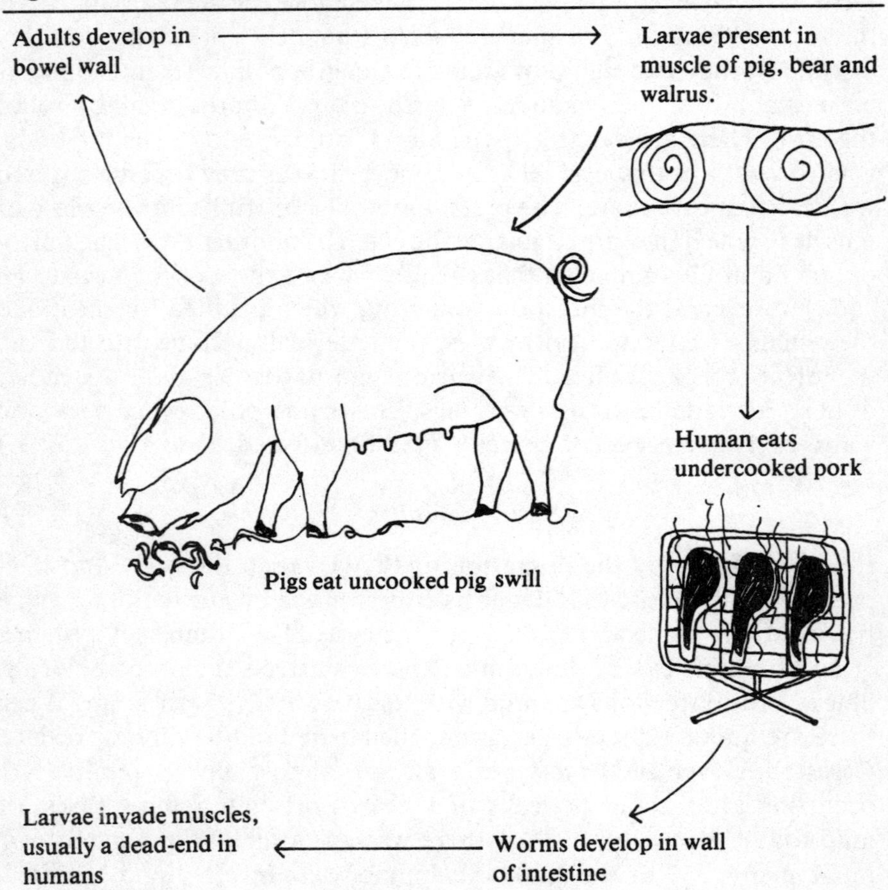

Worms introduced directly through the skin

Hookworms

Hookworms, are quite small, the largest measuring only about half an inch, but they appear in large numbers, living in the small intestines of man and other animals. They hang on by sucking a plug of the lining membrane of the intestine into their mouths and then tearing it with teeth or cutting plates; at the same time, they produce a substance that prevents the blood from clotting so that blood sucked from the host passes down the worm's food canal and out through its anus. It is estimated that 500 such worms could remove about half a pint of blood per day so that the anaemia accompanying heavy infection is not unexpected.

Life cycle

The life cycle is very simple. Eggs are laid by the female worm; these pass down the intestine of the host and are excreted in the stools. If they are deposited in a warm moist area, the eggs develop into larvae. These are capable of passing through the skin of unprotected feet with which they come in contact in their vicinity; in this way they cause a mild rash around the ankles, known as 'ground itch'. Within the body of the host they make their way by means of the blood to the heart and thence to the lungs. Here they break through the air-sacs are, coughed up and swallowed; they thus reach the intestine to develop into fully grown worms. (See Figure 12.6.)

Varieties

There are two main types of hookworm: *Necator americanus* (the American Murderer) and *Ancylostoma duodenale*. Both are found mainly in warm countries with a low level of hygiene, throughout Africa, Asia and South America. The former type was common in the USA earlier in the century and even today occurs commonly in Georgia and Kentucky. Mines and tunnels provide the warmth and moisture needed by the larval worm to survive. The building of the St Gotthard Tunnel in Switzerland brought together miners from many countries; hookworm affected most of the workers; when they returned to the Netherlands, Germany, Belgium and England, they took the worm back home with them and for a long time it was common in the Cornish tin mines. However, today the infection is no longer common in Britain and most of the USA.

Schistosomes

During and just after the Second World War there was a British military hospital at a little town near Cairo called Tel-el-Kebir. At the hospital

Figure 12.6 Hookworms

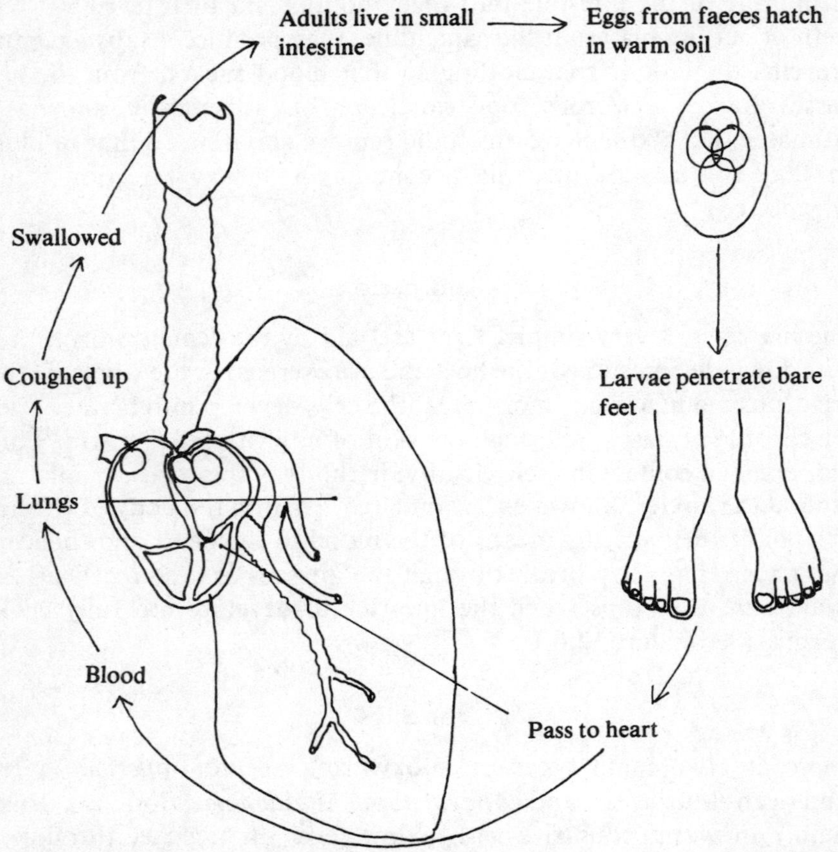

there was an officer's club known as the Bilharzia Club. 'Bilharzia' is the name given to the disease schistosomiasis caused by infection by *Schistosoma haematobium*, one of the three members of the group that infect man. The club emblem was a shield bearing a picture of an Egyptian dhow, a urine jar, a few drops of blood and an egg of the worm in question. This illustrates the importance of infection by this worm in that particular part of the world. Forty years later I visited Egypt again and I was told by a local pharmacist that, following the damming of the Nile, the incidence had increased. 'Practically every peasant suffers from it,' he said.

The worms

Three members of the schistosoma group affect man. *Schistosoma haemotobium* is common in most of Eastern Africa; *Sch. mansoni* is also widespread in Africa; while *Sch. japonicum* occurs only in the Far East and the Philippines. They are distinguishable easily by the shape of the eggs, which are a fraction of an inch in size, as seen under a microscope. The eggs of all types have spines but the situation of the spine differs with each type.

The worms themselves live in the large blood vessels surrounding the base of the bladder (*Sch. haematobium*) or around the rectum. The male has a split down the centre of his body and the female lies in this in a posture of continuous copulation ('schistosoma' means 'split body'). They are small worms, only about three quarters of an inch in length, but are believed to live in man for twenty to forty years. During this time large numbers of eggs are laid and, in order to complete the life cycle, these must escape from the human body. This is done by burrowing through either the bladder wall into the urine or the bowel wall into the faeces, according to the type of schistosome causing the infection.

In those parts of the world where the disease occurs, few people have the convenience of a convenience and make a convenience of the nearest collection of water; in this way the schistosome eggs reach the water.

Here the eggs hatch and motile larvae are set free. These can live for only a few hours unless they discover a snail of the correct sort. Within this snail multiplication takes place and, eventually, a different form of larva emerges which is able to swim and also to penetrate the skin of those rash enough to paddle or swim in that water. As with hookworms, the penetration by the larvae causes an itchy rash. They may also enter the body by the water being drunk. Within the body they soon reach the blood, which carries them all over the body, but only in the liver are they able to survive and mature. Once they have done so they pass to the veins round the bladder or the rectum, according to species, where they spend the rest of their lives. (See Figure 12.7.)

Two facts emerge from these life histories. The first is that snails can live in only still waters so that the effect of damming the Nile is to increase the number of snails and hence the incidence of the infection. The second is that the symptoms of the disease are caused by the efforts of the eggs to escape from the body.

Sch. haematobium and *Sch. mansoni* infect man only, but *Sch. japonicum* may infect cattle, horses, sheep, goats, pigs and other animals.

Figure 12.7 Schistosomiasis

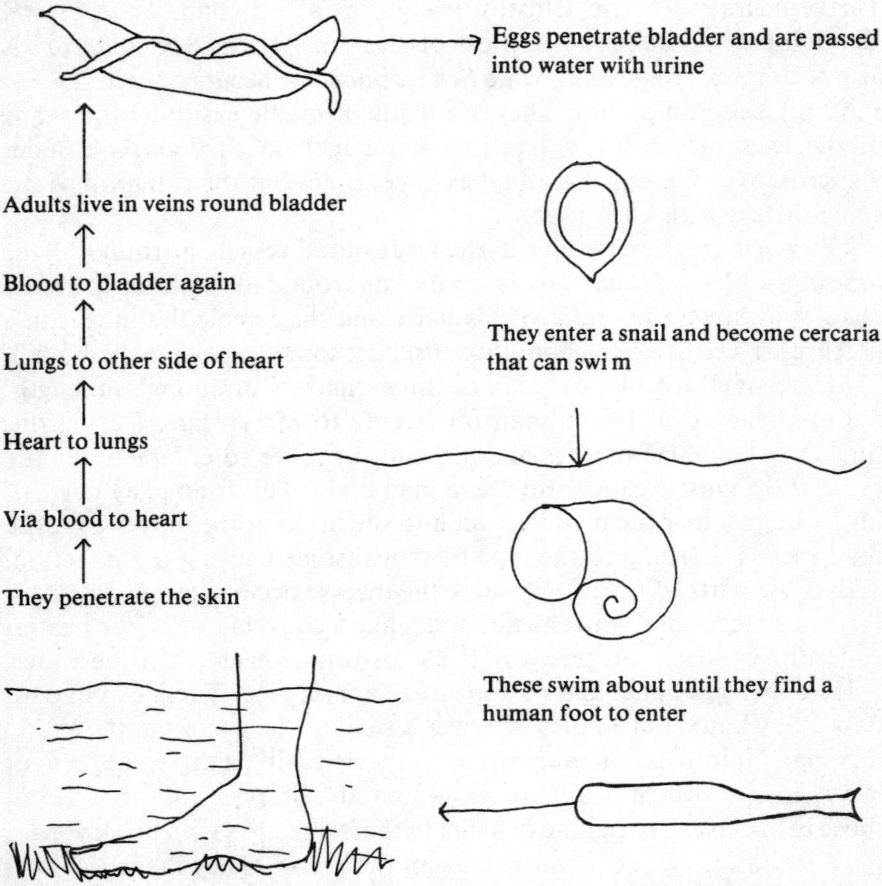

The disease of schistosomiasis

As the eggs penetrate the bladder or bowel wall they cause severe inflammation; where re-infection is continuous, as is usually the case in those who must work in or near infected water, this leads to replacement of the muscle of the bladder with thickened fibrous tissue and urine can no longer be 'squeezed' out of the bladder by muscle contraction. This will lead to chronic infection of the bladder, the ureters and the kidneys themselves; the result is further severe chronic illness and eventual death from infection or kidney damage. As we saw earlier, this parasite does not multiply in the human body so that a single infection, as suffered by a tourist, is not likely to cause serious damage—it is multiple infection that damages and kills.

Avoiding schistosomiasis

It is unwise for visitors to the Far East or Africa to paddle or bathe in areas of static water, except those specially treated for that purpose. As far as the local population are concerned, the fewer areas of static or slowly flowing water the better but this is counter to the principles of damming rivers to control flow and enhance power supply. Local people may be treated with drugs to prevent infection but this is expensive and must be repeated annually. The water may be treated with substances that will kill the snails. Copper sulphate has been used in the past but is being replaced by more sophisticated molluscicides.

Worms introduced by insects through the skin

Filaria

On new year's morning 1950, I awoke with a sore head and a dry mouth and then remembered that I had spent the previous night at a party given by the 'QAs'—the Queen Alexandra's Nursing Sisters attached to the No. 1 Military Hospital, Nairobi. However, on the table by my bed was a flask containing blood and some broken glass. Slowly the events of the previous night (or rather early morning) came back to me.

I had heard that we had, in the hospital, a patient with elephantiasis of the penis. This condition is caused by a small worm of the group known as 'filaria' (threadlike) blocking the lymphatic vessels. This prevents the lymphatic fluid from flowing back from the affected part and in turn leads to permanent swelling and thickening of the tissues. The degree of enlargement is quite astounding in untreated cases, even to the extent, in cases of elephantiasis of the scrotum, of the unfortunate victim having to wheel the affected part in front of him in a wheelbarrow! I remembered that I had gone to the ward armed with a syringe and a flask containing some broken glass (a primitive way of preventing the blood from clotting) and that I had asked the orderly: 'Wapi askari ya bora m'kubwa?' (which may be roughly translated from the Swahili as 'Where is the soldier with the enlarged penis?'). I was shown to a bed but the patient there strongly denied having that condition; however, he knew where the wanted patient was. The next patient also denied having the condition but knew where the patient in question was!

Eventually, a single file of patients with myself bringing up the rear discovered the wanted man from whom I must have taken blood into the flask before falling, exhausted, on my bed in my bungalow. Fortunately, I was able to see in the morning, under the microscope, the minute wormlike larvae of the worms responsible for the disease.

Now it must not be thought that my midnight excursion was due to suddenly remembering something I should have done during the day. This was far from being the case – it was done at this time because the larvae of the worm *Wucheria bancrofti* cannot be found in the blood during the day but appears there at night.

Filarial worms

There are a number of other filarial worms besides *W. bancrofti*, including one called *Loa loa*. They live for about ten years and either remain in the lymph glands or wander through the body. *Loa loa* has the distressing habit of occasionally crossing the conjunctiva, the transparent window of the eye. It is a very alarming experience and the worm can be seen wriggling across, taking about an hour to do so; strangely enough, apart from soreness for a few days no lasting harm is done. This is not the case, however, with another filarial worm, *Onchocerca volvulus*.

Life cycles

The small wormlike creatures seen in the blood are the first larvae of the adult worms and cannot cause infection. In order to do so they must mature within an insect. When the insect bites an uninfected person, some infective larvae escape from its 'mouth' and enter the puncture hole. Different types of worm rely on different insects: *Loa loa* on 'mango flies' in West Africa, *W. bancrofti* uses a variety of types of mosquito and *O. volvulus* uses black flies of the Simulium family, including one called *Simulium damnosum* – one gets the impression that the scientist who christened this fly had suffered severely from it before doing so! (See Figure 12.8.)

Onchocerca volvulus

While the adults of *W. bancrofti* and *Loa loa* are small worms, those of *O. volvulus* may be up to twenty inches in length. These worms live mainly in the tissue under the skin and produce nodules the size of a chestnut, containing a dozen or so tangled worms. The larval forms are present in the blood and also migrate through the tissues. They frequently enter the eye and when they die there they cause severe inflammation, often leading to blindness – *Onchocerciasis* the so-called 'river blindness'. This condition is a common cause of blindness, especially in Africa (tropical as well as the Sudan), in the Yemen and in South America.

Figure 12.8 Filarial worms

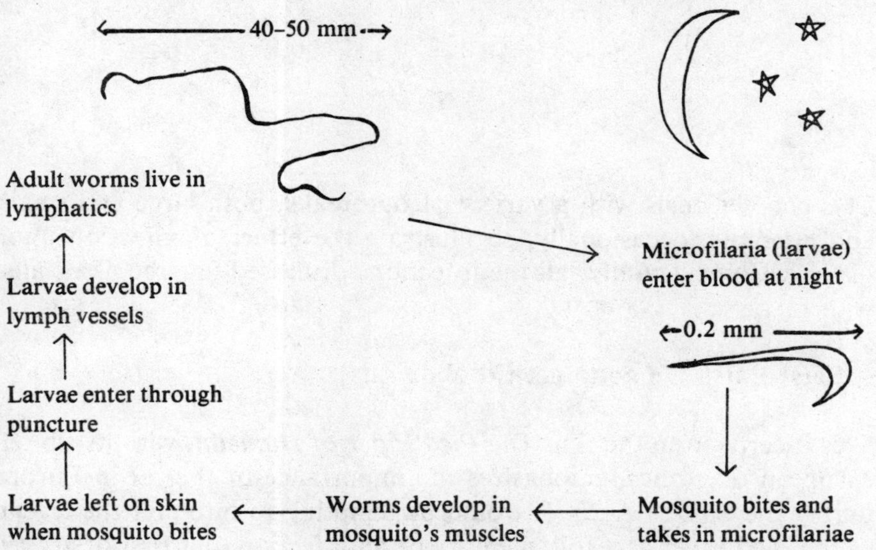

Avoiding filarial infestation

The incidence of these diseases can be reduced by attempting to kill the larvae of the insect vector. Slow release brickettes of DDT and other substances may be used. *Loa loa* infection can be prevented by the prophylactic use of drugs. Infection by filarial worms may be treated by various drugs but once the eye has been damaged by *O. volvulus*, drug treatment will not restore the sight, although corneal grafts may be successful.

THIRTEEN

Plagues and Other Epidemics

This chapter deals with a variety of outbreaks, both large and small, and attempts, occasionally, to illustrate the effect of infection upon history. Coincidentally, all the infections discussed may be associated with rats.

Rats! Rats! We gotta get rid o' de rats!

This excerpt from the film *The Pied Piper of Hamelin*, with its Mitteleuropean overtones, emphasizes the importance of the rat in Europe during the Middle Ages. It would be tempting to interpret the legend of the Pied Piper as a folk memory of an infection that first destroyed the rats and then the children but, unfortunately, the hypothesis will not fit. It seems more likely that the legend is a synthesis of two stories. One describes the miraculous elimination of rats from the city by a mediaeval rodent extermination officer of great proficiency. The other was based on the recruitment of German teenagers to the rich lands of eastern Europe, where the soil was fertile and labour was scarce; a country now known as Czechoslovakia, the western part of which was later to be 'liberated' by Hitler, the area was then known as Sudetenland.

Rats do not seem to have been present in Europe during classical times, arriving between AD 400 and 1100 (not a very precise dating). The first type to arrive was the black rat, an agile climber that was able to use mooring ropes to board ships, so that it frequently became seagoing. As it was the black rat that spread plague, its naval proclivities enabled it to carry the infection from country to country.

During the eighteenth century the Continent was invaded by the brown rat, which succeeded in replacing the black rat in all but a very few places, and this may have had something to do with the gradual disappearance of plague throughout Europe, which began at this time.

Rats carry (and transmit) many diseases, including the following: plague, typhus, trichinosis, haverhillosis, leptospirosis, foot and mouth disease, equine influenza and some strains of salmonella – an impressive list of infections but fewer than carried by dogs.

Plague

This word is often used to describe the widespread occurrence of something unpleasant; the Egyptians suffered a plague of frogs; we may suffer a plague of wasps or ants. Our grandchildren may be the plagues of our life and we refer to them as 'pests'. It therefore follows that 'plague' is a specific infectious disease caused by *Yersinia pestis*.

Plague is a disease of rodents and is passed from animal to animal by infected fleas. Occasionally, man is bitten by such infected fleas whose host has died or from whom they have departed for various reasons; in this case man develops plague. Occasionally, for reasons we do not understand (although recent work suggests a mutation in the plague bacillus as being the reason), pandemics of the disease occur. It is obvious that such outbreaks cannot occur unless many rats come into contact with many humans and generously share their fleas so that plague outbreaks in the Middle Ages and later depended largely on the heavy rat infestation of people's dwellings. It is highly unlikely that outbreaks of plague will occur in the Western world in view of the general level of rat control obtaining there. However, the situation in the Third World is different and, even in the West, conditions of war and famine could easily alter the situation radically.

The rat flea usually bites humans on the leg and the plague bacilli are carried upwards. The lymph glands of the groin attempt to delay their progress and become enlarged and painful. This swelling is known as a 'bubo' so that this type of plague is called 'bubonic'. Once past the lymph glands the organisms multiply rapidly and cause a severe septicaemia, killing the patient, often in a matter of hours. The mortality varies from 60 per cent to 90 per cent.

As the organisms multiply throughout the body, the lungs become infected if the patient survives long enough. As a result, before he dies, the patient may be coughing up large numbers of plague bacilli. In winter, especially in the Middle Ages, in order to keep warm it was necessary to restrict ventilation drastically. This resulted in airborne spread of the organism, causing 'pneumonic' plague which spreads rapidly and fatally.

Between epidemics

It would seem that, between epidemics, the plague bacillus is present in a variety of rodents and spread by their own special fleas. Thus, in the USA the infection may be present in ground squirrels, wood rats and prairie dogs as well as in chipmunks and marmots. Occasional bites experienced by humans from an infected flea result in the occurrence of a small number of cases of plague; thus, between 1905 and 1966 there were 115 cases of plague with 65 deaths in the USA. In South America the commonest reservoir is in the guinea-pig.

The organism was first introduced into South Africa in 1900 through rats from ships from South America; between 1919 and 1943 more than 900 outbreaks of plague have been recorded there, most of them small. In Mongolia and Manchuria marmots are the main carriers; these animals are sought after for their fur. Chinese or Russian hunters may disturb them during hibernation and consequently be bitten by their fleas, contracting bubonic plague, while in winter pneumonic plague may become epidemic. In many parts of the world plague occurs but is not reported. While the Americans were in Vietnam, they were surprised to discover over 5000 cases between 1955 and 1957 and the conditions in the country were such that there seemed little hope of eradicating the disease.

Apart from the latter finding, it does seem that plague today is a widespread disease of rodents, only occasionally affecting man; however, it may be the malignant genii in the bottle waiting to get out!

Earlier outbreaks of plague

Jehovah, in the Old Testament, appears to have used infectious disease, not only to help the Israelites defeat their enemies (in the same way that malaria helped the Allies defeat the Japanese during the Second World War) but also against his chosen people themselves when he felt they deserved chastisement. An episode in the Book of Samuel appears to describe an outbreak of bubonic plague. It seems that the Philistines inconsiderately captured the Ark of the Covenant, so that the Lord smote them with 'emerods in their secret parts'. Although the word 'emerod' sounds like the modern 'haemorrhoid', we have to remember that the translators of the Bible were trying to interpret an Aramaic word that meant only 'swelling'. Some have suggested that the infection was dysentery, causing an epidemic of 'prolapsed piles' as a result. It is more likely that the swellings were of the inguinal glands ('buboes') and it is interesting that the Philistines, when they made reparation, provided five 'golden emerods'. Neither piles nor buboes are articles of natural beauty and neither possess a characteristic recognizable shape when separated from their normal environment; it must have needed a Semitic Henry Moore or Barbara Hepworth to make a thing of beauty of their sculptures. Interesting, too, was the fact that with the five golden emerods came five golden mice! Were these in reality golden rats and did the Philistines know something about the spread of plague that did not become common knowledge until the twentieth century?

The Philistines returned the Ark of the Covenant to the Israelites and it arrived back near the village of Beth Shemesh; here the inquisitive inhabitants were said to have looked into it so that the Lord smote 50,070 of them 'with great slaughter' for their curiosity. It is tempting to think that the wily Philistines returned a few live and infected rats in the Ark together with the golden ones!

Plague in early times

The first great epidemic of what was recognized as being most probably bubonic plague was the Plague of Justinian, beginning in AD 540. This spread from the Far East, reaching Egypt and Palestine in its first year and then extending into Byzantium.

All ancient accounts of catastrophies, including plague, tend to gain in their repetition and may be elaborated by the story teller; after all, when we describe an accident we tend to emphasize its serious nature. 'Small earthquake in Wales. Little damage done' is the epitome of 'non-news' and a form of presentation favoured by few reporters. In the Middle Ages, spirits and ghosts were very real to the people so that we are not surprised to be told that: 'To many appeared phantoms in human forms. Those who were so encountered were struck a blow by the phantom and so contracted the sickness.'

The Plague of Justinian lasted until about 690 and, although at first the death rate was comparatively low, in the later days 5,000 to 10,000 people died daily. This long and serious calamity must have had a severe weakening effect on both Rome and Byzantium and at least brought forward the falls of these empires to the barbarians.

The Black Death

Plague has spread across the world on many occasions but for Britain the most terrible and influential visitation was the Black Death that arrived during the 1340s.

Early in that decade, a party of Italian merchants returning from the 7,000-mile silk route to China was attacked by Tartar bandits so that they took refuge in a fort called Caffa in the Crimea in southern Russia; in this fort they were besieged for three years. Toward the end of this period the Tartars were stricken by plague and had to raise the siege but, before doing so, they catapulted bodies of their colleagues who had died of plague over the battlements. Whether it was this quite creditable early attempt at germ warfare or the entry of a few non-aligned but infected rats into the fortress that introduced plague into the besieged party is not clear; but, when it was found that the Tartars had departed, the merchants took ship to Europe and carried the plague with them.

The first infections occurred in Genoa and the disease spread through Italy and Sicily; it reached Spain, France and Germany in June 1348 and by December was in northern Europe, entering England via Weymouth (then called Melcombe Regis) in August 1348. It then rapidly spread through England but took some time to reach Scotland. The Scots ascribed the sufferings of the English to their wickedness and congratulated themselves on their own immunity. But, when they seized the opportunity and they made a foray to the South, 'their joy turned to mourning as the sword of the wrath of God . . . scourged them in fury, smiting them no less than the English with abscesses and pustules'.

By the winter of 1349 the Black Death was over in Britain, by then having killed between one third and one half of the population.

The effects of the Black Death

It is difficult to imagine the situation in which half the population dies within a few months. Half one's relatives, children and friends die; half the doctors die, together with half the undertakers and coffin makers, so that the dead must be disposed of by mass burial in communal trenches, while, for the religious, there will not be priests available to administer last rites.

Such was the situation existing in Britain at that time and it had a profound effect on the morale of the survivors. Some turned, desperately, to religion; the flagellants marched, in large numbers, through the towns, chanting hymns and confessions and beating themselves unmercifully until the blood ran freely. Others decided to eat, drink and be merry, making use of the property and belongings of those who had died to live it up in a way they had never been able to do before.

The disruption of the economy, especially through the shortage of workers to harvest, process and transport food, led to famine in many parts, more so on the Continent, where sometimes cannibalism followed.

In a town in Germany a man and his two sons killed a pregnant woman. They cleaned the corpse and scraped the flesh from the bones; some of the flesh they pickled and some they took home to eat fresh, saying that 'they had found a pig by the roadside'. The family tucked in and in four days they were all dead—the woman had been heavily infected with plague when they killed her.

It was a great time for the 'heavy boys' of those days. In Italy the Becchini, or 'gravediggers', were employed to take people suffering from the infection to the plague hospitals. These gravediggers were mainly released criminals but also active entrepreneurs. Rich men were able to get rid of their enemies by bribing the gravediggers to take them by force to the plague hospitals; if not infected before, they rapidly became so in the hospitals. Later, with creditable initiative, the gravediggers took to breaking into the houses of the healthy and dragging husbands, wives or children to the plague hospitals if they were refused money.

The Black Death and English society

The population of England increased threefold between 950 and 1250 but then the situation began to change because, between about 1300 and 1500, there was a 'Little Ice Age' in Europe when the summers became wetter and colder and the harvests failed year after year. The existing tendency towards a decrease in population was greatly accelerated by the Black Death which halved, in one year, the number of workers available for tilling the fields.

At that time the feudal system was in full swing. The peasant held a strip or two of the lord's land for his own use and in exchange he was expected to cultivate the lord's demesne. The work on the lord's land was expected to be carried out at the appropriate time for the task (sowing, harvesting, etc.) so that the peasant was not able to work his own strips at the most important times. The halving of the population by the plague meant that there was more money available per head so that many peasants could now afford to pay their rent in *cash*; with this cash the lord was able to employ free labourers to work on his demesne—a revolutionary situation. At the same time, many of the younger peasants absconded, becoming free labourers in other parts of the country.

Because of the shortage of labourers, the workers were now in a position to negotiate with their employers and a scenario of almost modern dimensions evolved. The workers demanded more pay and went on strike if they did not get it; the government proclaimed a pay freeze and threatened to prosecute employers who paid their workers higher wages than before the Black Death; on occasions justices were chased from their courts by angry labourers—what today would be described as 'peaceful picketing'. Thus the Black Death led to a completely different relationship between the employer and the employee.

A further effect of the Black Death was that more land was turned over to sheep raising because this was not as labour intensive as the cultivation of the soil. This made the important English wool trade even more important. A more unlikely effect of the Black Death followed the high mortality among senior clergy in England. These, who were predominantly Norman and thus spoke French, had to be replaced at such short notice by local, English-speaking clerics. Thus English became the language of the Church and the State. If it had not been for the Black Death it is possible that French might be spoken as widely as English is today.

The further history of plague in Britain

After the Black Death, plague remained endemic in Britain, flaring up from time to time. Between 1500 and 1720 there were forty-five pandemics of plague but not all affected Britain. The most important outbreak after the Black Death was the Plague of London (which was not confined to that city) in 1665. Out of a population of half a million, London had up to 8,000 deaths a week. In 1666 the Great Fire of London destroyed a large part of the maze of rat-infested wooden buildings, which were replaced by buildings of brick and stone that were less penetrable by rats. This might explain the future freedom from plague enjoyed by London but does not account for the same freedom enjoyed by the rest of the country; perhaps the replacement of the black rat by the brown one played some part.

Epilogue

In 1910 there were four cases of rapidly fatal pneumonia in the village of Freston, near the river Orwell in Suffolk. The condition was so unusual that blood and sputum from the patients was sent to London for examination; *Y. pestis* was isolated from all specimens. This set the authorities thinking and they then remembered eight cases and six deaths at Shotley in 1906 and eight cases with five deaths at Trimley in 1909, both villages being only a few miles from Freston. As a result, a programme of trapping and examining rodents in the area was initiated and a small number of rats and hares was found to be infected with *Y. pestis*; continued monitoring found some infected animals in the vicinity as late as 1918.

Typhus

This infection, which was differentiated from typhoid fever only in the nineteenth century, is caused by small bacterium-shaped organisms known as 'rickettsiae'. Rickettsiae are named after Howard Ricketts, an American bacteriologist, who died in Mexico in 1910 from the infection while investigating its cause and showing that it could be spread by the body louse.

There are two types of typhus, caused by closely related strains of rickettsiae.

1. *Epidemic typhus* is spread from man to man by the body louse (and sometimes by the head louse). Its only mammalian host was believed, up to a few years ago, to be man but, recently, it has been shown that the disease also affects flying squirrels in the USA and is spread by squirrel fleas; in a few instances, humans living in houses visited by these squirrels have developed the disease. Epidemic typhus is a disease of war, poverty and dirt. It occurs mainly in colder countries where there is little incentive to remove the clothes regularly.
2. *Murine typhus* is a disease of rats and is spread by their fleas and also their lice. Man becomes infected only incidentally when bitten by an infected rat flea. The infection occurs mainly in South America and parts of Africa.

The disease

The organism spreads throughout the body and damages the walls of blood vessels; as the latter are present in all the organs of the body, damage may be widely distributed.

After an incubation period of ten to fourteen days the illness begins with headache, fever and vomiting. After about seven days a rash appears, caused by bleeding from the damaged skin blood vessels; the rash persists and darkens. Because the blood vessels are so damaged, the blood supply to parts that stick out may be restricted; this leads to gangrene, which may affect fingers, toes, the nose and the genitalia, any or all of which may drop off. The fatality rate depends on age, varying from nil in young children to 100 per cent in people over sixty.

In some parts of the world, e.g. Mexico, both types of typhus have existed together for centuries.

Brill–Zinsser disease

American doctors were surprised to observe mild attacks of typhus affecting middle-aged Polish and Russian immigrants in New York in the absence of wider outbreaks. It was eventually shown that these illnesses were recurrences of infection in people who had been infected many years before in their native lands. Thus the rickettsiae are capable of existing for many years in people who have been infected but causing no symptoms.

Some effects of typhus

The Plague of Athens could have been typhus, although it could as easily have been ergot poisoning. The disease was common in Britain throughout the Middle Ages right up to the end of the eighteenth century. It was common in gaols and known as 'gaol fever'. Visitors to prisons almost always carried nosegays in an attempt to discourage the typhus agent from infecting. Possibly because of the prevalence of the disease in prisoners, there were a number of 'Black Assizes' in the sixteenth century when a large proportion of those present in court, including the judges, became ill and died. Another explanation for these judicial outbreaks might be the carriage of infected lice by spectators. In at least one case the infection and mortality was neatly confined to persons on one side of the court. It seems possible that, on a swelteringly hot day, one of the spectators in the gallery may have taken off his wig to fan himself and, unwittingly, despatched a volley of deadly lice on to the assembly below. Lice were quite happy to live in wigs, as well as live hair, as Samuel Pepys knew to his discomfort.

Later on, during the English Civil War, typhus infected soldiers on both sides with impartiality so that any effect on the outcome cannot be measured.

In the eighteenth century typhus killed rather more people in Britain than did smallpox and there were more Black Assizes. In the nineteenth century the disease was rife in Ireland. During the years of famine caused by the failure of the potato crop, between 1847 and 1851 it was estimated that nearly 1 million people died. Of these, many died of typhus and the infection was still present in a small way in Ireland early in the twentieth century. At the time of the famine over 2 million Irishmen emigrated to the USA, so that typhus must be one of the causes of the marked Irish element in that country. In England, in the north-west counties near the port of Liverpool there were about 10,000 cases in 1847–8, presumably spreading from Ireland.

It was during and after the First World War that typhus came into its own. It appears to have broken out in Serbia in November 1914, affecting both the Serbs and their 70,000 Austrian prisoners. Of the 400 doctors available nearly all contracted the infection dying from it and in six months 150,000 people died, including half the Austrian prisoners. The presence of this outbreak prevented the Austrians from attacking early and must have had a profound effect on the course of operations in the East and, indirectly, in the West, possibly influencing the balance in the war. Did typhus win the First World War?

The disease flourished as the war progressed. In Russia there were 100,000 cases in the first year of the war, rising to 164,000 during the second year. After this the incidence increased and it is probable that, between 1917 and 1921, there were 25 million cases with 2.5 to 3 million deaths in Russia alone. There were also many cases in the Baltic states and Poland.

In the Second World War typhus broke out in Naples in 1943–4 but, for the first time, it was possible to deal effectively with such an outbreak, using insecticides (DDT) and by vaccinating military personnel.

Today typhus is an uncommon disease in most countries but may occur sporadically in those where rat infestation is common. It is susceptible to antibiotics such as tetracycline or chloromycetin. In conditions of war, with poverty, dirt and dislocation of services, it could easily return.

Leptospiral infection (Weil's disease)

One day in the spring of 1948 two NCOs attached to the Queen Alexandra's Military Hospital in Surrey disappeared unofficially for a binge at the local pub. Characteristically, the hospital had been built on a swamp and the ditches surrounding it contained water and were overrun with rats.

When the convivial soldiers returned, they fell into the waterlogged ditches because of the darkness and other circumstances. They became soaked and possibly even swallowed (accidentally, of course) some of the water contained in the ditches.

About ten days later both became suddenly ill with severe headaches, pains in the joints and muscles, fever and shivering. A few days later still, both developed jaundice, which became progressively darker. Examination of their blood showed a great increase in those white cells associated with infection and this proved that they had contracted infection with leptospira, a condition often known as Weil's disease.

The organism and the illness

The condition is caused by a spiral organism resembling the one that causes syphilis but having looser and untidier spirals. It is known as *Leptospira icterohaemorrhagiae* and it is associated with rats. It caused infection in the trenches in the First World War and later in the rat-infested coal mines of East Lothian in Scotland. Although found in most parts of the world, it became known in Britain as an occupational hazard of sewer workers and also affected the Aberdeen fish-cleaning lassies. It is also a hazard to inexpert canoeists and drunks who fall into canals. Up to 45 per cent of rats have been found infected in areas where the disease occurs; both the black and the brown rat are involved.

The disease is, fortunately, fairly rare today. Fewer than one hundred cases occur each year in Britain, although it is officially regarded as an occupational disease.

A related organism, *Leptospira canicola*, infects dogs and can be passed from them to humans, in whom it causes a mild form of meningitis.

Ratbite fever and related infections

When rats were commonly present in human habitations, infections following their bites were not uncommon, as happens with leptospirosis discussed above. Two separate organisms seem to cause ratbite fever.

One type of infection is caused by *Spirillum minus*, which is a sort of sawn-off spirochoete, possessing only one or two coils. Following a bite from a rat, cat or other animal, one to three weeks later there is a sudden onset of fever accompanied by a dark red rash. The condition clears up after a few days but recurs a few days after that. Most of the cases described occurred before the days of antibiotics and a mortality rate of 2 per cent to 10 per cent was described. Today, it seems certain that prompt treatment with antibiotics would bring about a rapid cure.

The second type of ratbite fever is caused by an organism with the awesome name of *Streptobacillus moniliformis*, which simply means 'the bacillus that forms chains and may be mistaken for a yeast'. The organism is present in the throats of most rats and also some other animals, including turkeys. About ten days after the bite there is a sudden onset of illness, with a splitting headache, fever, shivering and pains in the joints and muscles. A little later, a rash appears in the form of redness and blisters over the hands, feet and face. Once again, the illness may appear to clear up but then recurs a few days later.

Haverhill fever

In January 1926 there was an outbreak of illness in the town of Haverhill, Massachusetts, USA, consisting of about sixty cases. There was severe headache, fever, muscle pains and a rash on the hands, feet and face. The mortality rate was about 4 per cent. Eventually, *Streptobacillus moniliformis* was isolated from many of these patients but *there was in no case a history of a rat bite*! It was assumed that the infection originated from milk contaminated by infected rat urine but the evidence was flimsy.

Haverhill fever in Britain

In February 1983 I was asked to look into an outbreak of illness in a girls' boarding school. It was a well-run convent school with 500 pupils, of whom 370 were boarders. There was also a large staff and a community of elderly, retired nuns.

The illness

At the beginning of the outbreak a small number of girls had suddenly been smitten with splitting headaches, fever, joint and muscle pains and shivering. A day or so later a rash developed on the feet, hands and face. The distribution of the rash resembled that of smallpox but there the resemblance ended. Many of the girls were quite ill and, as the days passed, more and more went down with the disease, as did also some of the elderly nuns in the community.

Specimens of all types were taken from the girls for laboratory examination but all were negative. We strongly suspected some type of virus infection but both virus culture and electron microscopy showed no sign of any virus. We also cultured the blood but found no organisms present—this seems to have been an occasion when my own laboratory was found wanting. A few of the girls recovered sufficiently to be sent home but then promptly relapsed. Some had their blood cultured by other laboratories and it was discovered that two girls had *Streptobacillus moniliformis* in their blood! (The microbiologists concerned, having made this splendid breakthrough, then blotted their copybooks by describing the outbreak and its causation, even though none had ever ventured within miles of the school—an occupation known as 'armchair epidemiology'.)

This, then, was an outbreak of haverhillosis, ratbite fever without ratbites—the school authorities were rightly offended when the condition was loosely referred to as 'ratbite fever'.

In all 304 persons were affected, 43 per cent of the total population of the school. Remembering the mortality rate of 4 per cent in the 1926 outbreak, we were very apprehensive, dreading the deaths of up to twelve patients; however, there were no deaths and all those infected made a complete recovery, possibly because of the use of antibiotics and also the devoted nursing, especially on the part of the sister in charge of the hospital.

The source of the infection

Where did the infection originate? The 1926 outbreak was believed to be caused by milk, which was where we first looked. The school had its own dairy and, up until the outbreak, unpasteurized milk was used by the school; any residue of milk produced by the dairy was sent for pasteurization and sale elsewhere. This at first seemed to suggest a milk-spread origin. However, inspection of the dairy (which had by now begun to pasteurize *all* its milk) showed no possible situation under which the milk could have been contaminated by rats. Rats were said to have been seen on the school premises but none were seen by us during the investigation; the nuns were not successful in trapping any but one offered to try to shoot one for me with an air rifle!

In the end a statistical approach was made to the problem. All members of the population were asked to fill in a questionaire on their eating and drinking habits and these were considered in the light of whether infection occurred or not.

It was found that there was a strong association between infection and the drinking of tap water but no strong association with milk drinking.

At that time there were two supplies of water to the school, a chlorinated mains supply and a supply from a spring. The spring water passed through an area where rats had been seen so that contamination could have taken place and this was assumed to have been the case.

These investigations cannot be thought of as conclusive, since they leave a large question unanswered; what volume of infected rat urine would be needed to contaminate the water, remembering how much that urine would be diluted, to such an extent as to cause infection to over 300 people? It would seem to require a synchronized effort on the part of a vast number of rats.

As with the outbreak of Legionnaire's disease in Philadelphia, this outbreak taught us that old-fashioned bacteria are still capable of causing large outbreaks of infection that may be difficult to identify.

FOURTEEN

The Control of Infection

In ancient days

Since the beginning of civilization methods of controlling infectious diseases have been sought. Moses was fairly late in the field, the Egyptians having preceded him by many hundreds of years, but at least he was thorough. The Egyptians were, for instance, insistent that meat should be cooked as soon as the animal had been killed and, similarly, in the Bible, Joseph orders his servants to 'slay and make ready' meat for his brothers. In the wilderness the Israelites obeyed specific and detailed laws intended to protect them from infection among other things; laws that today are obsolete in function but still adhered to by orthodox Jews.

In the Book of Leviticus, the Lord instructed Moses and Aaron how to discern leprosy (not the leprosy we know today, but an acute infectious dermatitis that seemed common in those days and in that particular location). The patient was ordered to keep himself isolated and to report to the priest every week; when the eruption had cleared up he was allowed back into the community. In some cases it was recommended that the garments of the patient should be burned, a practice that has been applied to some infections as late as the present century. Treatment appeared to be a mixture of therapeutics and magic, using cedar wood, scarlet (?), oil and hyssop (the latter probably chosen for its aromatic smell, using the same criteria that is often used in choosing disinfectants today!). Birds were sacrificed at the same time, these probably being a sort of consultation fee.

Precautions were also taken against venereal diseases, including the washing of the penis and of any garment soiled by semen (or urethral discharge?). Women with vaginal discharges, especially at times other than those of their normal periods, were regarded as unclean and had to undergo purification; the price for a certificate of good health was two pigeons. Casual sex with women, especially of other 'races' was forbidden.

It was insisted that, after killing, an animal should be drained of blood, this possibly enhancing the keeping qualities of the meat in a hot country without the benefit of refrigerators. A list of proscribed animals for meat was drawn up, including camels and pigs; the latter were no doubt included to avoid tapeworms and other parasites such as trichinella. Rabbits were also forbidden and, although 'straightforward' fish were permitted, less obvious seafood, including shellfish, was not.

Contaminated vessels were to be broken and discarded, while water supplies that had been contaminated were condemned unless free flowing. One regulation warned against eating 'the kid seethed in its mother's milk'. This was interpreted to mean that milk and meat should not be included in the same dish. When, about thirty years ago, it was discovered that a formula baby food contained an added protein supplement to boost the nutritive properties of the dried milk, this product was deemed by orthodox Jewish mothers to be unclean in view of the above exhortation.

The Middle Ages

As early as the seventh century the danger of mass movements of infected persons was understood, when, during an outbreak of plague in France, a group of 'security guards' was stationed between the plague-ridden district of Provence and the 'clean' area of Cahors. This physical prevention of the spread of infected persons has been used so often that it has been given the respectable name of cordon sanitaire and was used most recently by the Sudan during the outbreak of Ebola fever.

The great increase in long distance maritime ventures in the Middle Ages greatly increased the chances of serious infection, especially plague, reaching Europe. The theory of the incubation period was understood so that it became the habit to incarcerate ships and their crews for a period of time, during which any incubating infection would have shown itself. At first the period of thirty days was used but it was felt more respectable to use the period of time spent, at different times, by Jesus and by Moses in the desert; hence, forty days became the prescribed period and this gave rise to the term 'quarantine', from the Italian word for forty. After this period the ship was given a clean bill of health which protected it from further incarceration before voyaging to the East again. Although the process was extended for use in situations of suspected yellow fever, smallpox and cholera as well as plague, today the practice is rarely used and the word quarantine is confined to the very necessary process of detaining in high security kennels dogs imported from abroad, in an effort to avoid the importation of rabies; the period has been extended to six months.

The general public has always had its terror of infection and used its own methods of avoiding it, for instance the use of nosegays of flowers in prisons in order to avoid typhus. In 1973 there was an outbreak of yellow fever that *really* decimated the population of Philadelphia – it actually killed 10 per cent. During the outbreak it was said that 'many shut themselves in their houses and were afraid to walk the streets . . . People hastily shifted their course at the sight of a hearse . . . Many never walked on footpaths but went into the middle of the street to avoid passing by houses wherein people had died'. It is tempting to be amused at these naive precautions but we should bear in mind that, in recent times, people have contracted Legionnaire's disease (and died from it) in London merely by walking into or by buildings where cooling towers or air conditioning systems were contaminated.

Infections and hospitals

Hospitals in the West originated mainly in religious institutions, especially convents. (Hence the title 'Sister' for senior nurses, especially those in charge of a ward. The term 'Matron' is unlikely to have been derived from this source and probably reflected the work of the wife of a 'master' of a workhouse. I worked for a time in what was called a general hospital but which was known to the locals as the 'Werk 'ouse'; the then matron was the widow of the former workhouse master.)

For a long time hospitals hardly recognized the possibility of infection occurring within their walls. During the Crimean War it was said that wounded soldiers begged not to be sent to the hospital at Scutari because they knew that they were more likely to die there from dysentery than from their untreated wounds; we have also seen the situation in maternity hospitals in the middle of the nineteenth century. In the Hôtel Dieu in Paris (one of the many religious hospitals founded under this name during the seventeenth century, there were often as many as five patients to a bed and, when one of them died, the body was often not removed for twenty-four hours. In recent times it was the practice in British hospitals to retain the same blankets on a hospital bed no matter what the condition of patients passing through those beds; the only circumstance under which the blankets were changed was when a patient died in them! Although she poured scorn on the germ theory of infection, Florence Nightingale made a remark to the effect that the least we can ask from hospitals is that they do the patient no harm. This has been far from the truth until recent years.

We have seen that a patient's immunity is seriously damaged when the continuity of his tissues (especially skin) is interrupted, so that surgical and burns patients and newly delivered mothers are at greatest risk of infection. In recent years surveys have been carried out, particularly by the Public Health Laboratory Service, to find out exactly what proportion of patients in hospital developed infection there. It was found, in 1960, that nearly 10 per cent of patients admitted to hospitals developed an infection. Much research was carried out to discover the sources of such infection and it was found that, frequently, the patient brought the organism in with him. This led to the practice of trying to 'clean' patients before operating when there was time (i.e. in cases of 'cold' surgery). Much information about the spread of infection within hospital was obtained and the construction of subsequent hospitals has reflected this, although there had already been a movement away from large open wards to wards with blocks of 2- and 4-bed rooms. (In my time at an old-fashioned general hospital there was usually only a single single-bedded sideward to each open ward and this was usually occupied by a terminally ill patient, a member of staff or a clergyman). Thus, although infection still occurs in hospitals, case-to-case spread has been reduced. Most modern outbreaks are from single sources, be they food poisoning or Legionnaire's disease.

Fever hospitals

Hospitals built specifically to house cases of infectious disease began to appear mainly in the nineteenth century. The period from 1880 to 1930 was the heyday for the building of hospitals for patients suffering from tuberculosis, known as 'sanatoriums' or, more colloquially, as the 'sanny'. These served a double purpose: they protected the public by the isolation of infectious cases of tuberculosis and they provided an environment and regime designed to arrest the tuberculous process at work in the patient's lung. Patients spent long periods, measured in years, in the sanatorium where, in addition to good food and fresh air, they occasionally underwent operations designed to rest or even remove the affected lung.

The situation has now changed completely; because of the emergence of suitable antibiotics and similar substances, tuberculosis is now, if not rare, certainly unusual. Within a period measurable in hours from the onset of the action of the antibiotic, the patient ceases to cough up live tubercle bacilli and hence is no longer a menace to his fellows. Today, it is mainly the elderly man with a chronic cough (often labelled a smoker's cough) who is liable to be suffering from undiagnosed tuberculosis and capable of conveying it to his grandchildren; all chronic coughs must be investigated.

During the period when smallpox visited Britain on a large scale, several smallpox hospitals were built. These were high security hospitals, located far away from towns and equipped in such a way as to minimize the chances of the organism escaping. Now that smallpox has been eradicated (the last 'natural' case appearing in Somalia in October 1977, although two further laboratory infections occurred later), these hospitals are no longer used but could be reopened if a new and highly contagious infection should appear in Britain.

During the same period fever hospitals (more formally 'Infectious Diseases Hospitals') began to appear. Many of these were partly purpose-built but also retained some wards from an earlier phase of life. I worked for some years in the early 1940 in a bright and busy little fever hospital in north-east England. We had an isolation block that would have compared well with modern ones; single rooms with their own bathroom and toilet, absolutely ideal for nursing infectious cases. However, several of the other wards dated from the First World War and were eminently unsuitable. We had two big wards usually full of diphtheria cases and another containing scarlet fever patients. Scarlet fever is caused by haemolytic streptococci and several types may be responsible; within that large ward cross infection with different types occurred, just as if the patients were suffering from quite different infections, so some of them developed ear infections and others more serious complications.

About twenty years ago the habit of keeping cases of infectious disease in special fever hospitals began to be abandoned. Instead new hospitals were built with isolation blocks similar to that described above. There were several reasons for this change, the most important being the great reduction in important infectious disease cases. Thus diphtheria and poliomyelitis were practically eradicated and scarlet fever became much reduced in incidence; these were the diseases that had taken up so much room in the open wards of the old fever hospitals. There were also reductions in the incidence of dysentery and of typhoid fever (it was rarely necessary to admit to hospital cases of infection due to other members of the salmonella group). Another reason was that, of the infectious diseases remaining, quite a few were no longer infectious in practice. Thus, with almost the whole population immunized against poliomyelitis, the risk of a case causing an infection is very remote. Most cases of meningitis are not infective and the same is true for cases of glandular fever. Other conditions that need to be admitted might be susceptible to the action of antibiotics, so that the period of infectivity of such cases might be very short indeed after the onset of treatment. Yet another reason was that, with the diminution of cases of infection that needed admission to hospital, it was no longer cost-effective to keep open large fever hospitals. It then became a matter of deciding whether to leave open only a small number of such hospitals, causing great inconvenience to many of the patients and their visitors or whether to integrate their beds into general hospitals. Finally, cases of infection frequently need treatment other than by the physician. Thus, a woman suffering from puerperal infection might need the services of an obstetrician or a surgeon and cases of poliomyelitis might need active physiotherapy as early as possible in convalescence.

Epidemiology—field work in infectious diseases

In 1868 there was a large outbreak of typhoid fever in Terling, a small Essex village. Of the 900 inhabitants, about 300 became infected and over thirty died. Although such outbreaks were not uncommon in the Britain of the mid nineteenth century, the Local Government Board (which was by no means a 'local' organization, but the forerunner of the Department of Health) sent down to investigate one of their staff, Dr Robert Thorne Thorne. He wrote a report to the Privy Council suggesting how the outbreak had occurred and made suggestions to prevent it happening in the future. Dr Thorne was an early career epidemiologist, as opposed to Doctors Snow and Budd, the one an anaesthetist and the other a physician, who had, somewhat earlier, elucidated the spread of cholera and typhoid fever respectively.

From this time we find full-time epidemiologists emerging. In 1846 the first Medical Officer of Health (MOH) in history had been appointed, for Liverpool, and this was in response to the cholera epidemics that had caused so many deaths in Britain and which led to the Public Health Act of 1848. Up to 1858 about thirty-five more MOsH were appointed, while, in 1872, a new Public Health Act divided the country into a number of districts and required each to appoint its own

MOH. At first these were carried out part time by general practitioners (Dr W. Gimson Gimson, who looked after the victims of the Terling fever, later became MOH for Witham, where his practice was situated). Later the post became full time and the MOH became an officer of the local authority. The MOH was responsible, with the help of his sanitary inspector, for investigating outbreaks of infection in his district and, up until the beginning of the Second World War, he was often the only epidemiologist available locally.

The National Health Service Act 1946

The National Health Service Act of 1946 took away the clinical activities of the MOH (he had hitherto been in clinical charge of patients in the fever hospitals) but left him with responsibility for vaccination and other preventive medicine. The Act effectively divided the medical profession into three groups: general practitioners responsible for what is now called 'primary care' of patients; hospital doctors, who dealt with those patients needing hospital treatment; and public health doctors, including MOsH and their staff. The MOH was still responsible for the epidemiology of his district and, in theory, hospitals were part of that district; however, such was the schism caused by the Act that MOsH were regarded by many hospital doctors as being practically non-medical and were frequently not welcomed on hospital premises.

The reorganization of the National Health Service in 1974

In 1974 the National Health Service was reorganized and the MOH disappeared, to be replaced by the District Medical Officer, one of a new breed of Community Physicians. By now the Sanitary Inspector had disappeared, being replaced by the Public Health Inspector; the latter, since he was divorced from the Health Authority, was a chief officer of the local authority in his own right (requests from such officers quite often reached my laboratory asking me to send all pertinent results to *their* offices rather than that of the MOH or community physician; this could not be done because many of the reports were subject to medical confidentiality). The Public Health Inspector was finally replaced by the Environmental Health Officer who, in general, appears to act and advise with very little medical support.

The District Medical Officer took over the responsibility for all the public health medicine in his district. This was usually delegated to a Medical Officer (Environmental Health), whose job it was to advise the local authority when necessary, presumably through the Environmental

Health Officer. These latter medical officers were referred to, for some reason, as 'proper officers'; there is no evidence that they are more (or less) proper than any other community physicians.

The Public Health Laboratory Service

The functions of laboratories in controlling infection

In order to control infectious disease it was first important to define the size and nature of the problem. This involved the setting up of bacteriology laboratories (the description 'microbiological' arrived later) in order to determine what organisms cause the majority of infections to be controlled. Many infectious diseases may be diagnosed with a 90 per cent chance of being correct, merely by history taking and examination. The remainder which possess few distinctive symptoms or signs, especially those formerly referred to as 'continued fevers', need laboratory assistance for diagnosis. Today, the laboratory has two additional functions. First, it can type the organisms isolated. There are several types of *Salm. typhi* and any single outbreak would be expected to be caused by a single type; in this way, outbreaks can be 'sorted out' and cases of illness associated with suspect foods, etc., with some degree of correctness. The second function is to determine the sensitivity of the organism to antibiotics. Although a prudent clinician will treat his patient with a usually reliable antibiotic, he will take a specimen for laboratory examination before starting treatment; it will be unwise for him to assume that the 'usual' antibiotic will be effective in every case, as so many antibiotic resistant strains have emerged in recent years.

Bacteriological laboratories before 1939

In 1937 there were a fair number of bacteriological laboratories in England and Wales but these were very unevenly distributed and few were involved in public health work. There were a few 'municipal laboratories', run by the larger cities and a few in London, but the majority were in the large corporations of the North and Midlands. Many local authorities provided laboratories for special purposes, such as tuberculosis or venereal disease work, but few carried out other duties. Many hospitals away from the large cities had no facilities for bacteriology whatsoever (in the mid 1940s when I was working in Middlesbrough, although there were three general hospitals, one maternity hospital and one very active fever hospital, there was not a single pathology department of any kind in the whole town!).

Where bacteriology laboratories *did* exist, there was rarely any communication between them, while the only national estimate of infectious diseases was produced by the Ministry of Health from reports from the MOsH mainly derived from notifications from general practitioners, almost entirely unsupported by laboratory findings (in my own time I have been tempted to investigate the effect of altitude on the prevalence of measles, only to find that the medical practice at the top of the hill notified all their cases while those in the valley notified none).

The Emergency Public Health Laboratory Service

In 1938 it seemed certain that Britain was on the threshold of war. Many doctors had seen, during the First World War, the effect of movement of population, disruption of sewerage systems and contamination of water supplies on the incidence of infection. Many had seen the large outbreaks of typhus in eastern Europe and had been struck by the number of deaths and the amount of distress resulting. This sort of thing, it was believed, could now happen to Britain, especially England. Most existing public health laboratories were sited in large towns, just those that might provide the most popular targets for enemy bombers. There was always the threat, remote though it was, of bacteriological warfare. It seemed necessary to strengthen the bacteriological services in the south of England, siting many of the laboratories away from large towns.

These matters had been considered as early as 1934 and in 1936 a subcommittee was set up of the, today, somewhat archaic-sounding Committee on Imperial Defence. The subcommittee recommended that an emergency public health service be set up. The word 'bacteriological' was never used because of its association with bacteriological warfare which, although unlikely to occur, was a source of worry, to say the least, to many uninformed people.

Professor Topley, of the London School of Hygiene, had been in Serbia in 1915 and had seen the ravages of typhus there. He stimulated the British Medical Research Council to set up a committee of medical administrators and bacteriologists to look into the setting up of a 'civilian bacteriological service to operate in time of war'. It was eventually decided to set up a network of emergency laboratories in the south of England, to be staffed by workers from leading teaching and research establishments. It was also recommended that the professors of bacteriology in the six universities in the Midlands and the North should prepare local schemes. Much apparatus was put aside, workers, including technical staff, were chosen and suitable (at least fairly suitable) buildings were earmarked as laboratories (five out of ten near London were on school premises). On 26 August 1939, members of staff reported to their posts and, when war was declared on 3 September, most of the laboratories were ready for action.

Thus, there came into existence the Emergency Public Health Laboratory Service (EPHLS). From the beginning it was an integrated service, with directors to each laboratory and 'central' laboratories. The latter were to support the 'area' laboratories, to provide services that were not suitable to be carried out on the periphery (usually on grounds of costs and manpower) and to supply locum staff from time to time.

In order to report progress a monthly bulletin was inaugurated and this was later incorporated into the clumsily titled *Bulletin of the Ministry of Health and the Public Health Laboratory Service*. The *Bulletin* both described outbreaks and new laboratory methods. Even later we were still in an era of 'do-it-yourself'. I once applied for a photo-electric colorimeter (a very expensive item at that time, costing about £200) and a bottle of buffer tablets costing a few shillings; I received a letter from the supplies department of the Service granting me the colorimeter but also saying that 'in the opinion of the Director of the Service a laboratory director should be able to make up his own buffer solutions'! Obviously, the director's time was of little value. I mention this because, in the *Bulletin* at about this time, there appeared a 'recipe' for making a machine for continuously turning a tissue-culture flask – out of Meccano!

From the very beginning the laboratory directors were required to send to headquarters a list of all findings of significance. The reports were collated and edited and the edited version sent out a week later to all laboratories as the *Weekly Summary of Laboratory Returns*; this was an invaluable source of information on the geography of infection in England and Wales. In 1954 this system was extended to all hospital bacteriology laboratories in England and Wales so that, since then, a more complete and accurate account of infection throughout the country has been available.

Those who remember the war years will recall that for the first few months we enjoyed what came to be called the 'phoney war', during which very little happened; later came the Battle of Britain and the Blitz and, although much damage was done, it was never sufficient to cause epidemics. The only movement of population of any size was the evacuation of children from more vulnerable areas to the North and Midlands and this caused no public health problems, apart from the odd extra visitor in the hair of some of the young evacuees. The laboratories of the EPHLS were able to turn their hands to more mundane subjects than the stemming of epidemics (one middle-aged medical microbiologist, a retired army officer with no experience of 'real' medicine for twenty years, found himself in charge of a community of pregnant evacuees).

However, the local MOsH were grateful for the presence of these laboratories. They could now obtain laboratory confirmation of their clinical diagnoses of conditions such as typhoid fever and were able to confirm the diagnosis of diphtheria with something more specific than the Infectious Diseases Hospital matron's sense of smell. They were also able to carry out their investigations into outbreaks of infection far more precisely and accurately. The laboratories were also able to monitor samples of milk and water from the consumer's angle.

No new system is immediately acceptable to all and the EPHLS was no exception. Many private laboratories depended for their living on the fees for examining milk and water specimens; this problem was solved by the Service examining only specimens as they reached the consumer. Another problem occurred when a hospital already had a bacteriologist; the latter might be very suspicious that the EPHLS man might wish to poach on his preserves. One of my EPHLS colleagues described, many years ago, how he and his hospital counterpart would sit and glare at each other from their respective laboratories.

Work of the Emergency Public Health Laboratory Service

During the war years, in the absence of any of the emergencies it had been set up to counter, the EPHLS gradually increased its scope and volume of work. It sorted out a number of outbreaks of typhoid fever; in 1939 there were 1500 notifications. It also devised a method of 'fingerprinting' strains of *Salm. typhi* so that outbreaks could be more clearly differentiated. It provided a service for the rapid diagnosis of diphtheria; in 1941 there were over 8,000 isolations. School outbreaks of diphtheria and dysentery were investigated, with healthy carriers of the former being looked for. Food poisoning outbreaks were investigated; these increased in number markedly during the war years and this was ascribed partly to better recognition and partly to the increasing tendency to eat out, a practice rare before the war (at one time the meat ration was to the value of six new pence so that eating, out especially at the 'British Restaurant'—the name given to members of a chain of simple cafeterias organized by the government, where a filling meal could be obtained at little cost-stretched the rations considerably). Whooping cough was studied and the possibility of obtaining a vaccine against the infection was explored.

The 1946 Act and the laboratory service

When the Bill for this Act came under discussion in 1944, it was recommended that there should be incorporated the proposal to set up a National Public Health Laboratory Service for England and Wales (Scotland has always relied mainly on its university laboratories for its public health services). In consequence the new service, now known as the Public Health Laboratory Service (PHLS), became a permanent feature on the health scene when the Act received assent in November 1946.

The Public Health Laboratory Service

A headquarters building was set up at the former Government Lymph Establishment at Colindale in north London. Here, there eventually came many of the special 'reference laboratories', each with its own sphere of interest, able to collate information about its speciality and also able to take investigations somewhat further than was practicable in the area laboratories. It was originally planned that there would be seventy laboratories in the Service; but this figure was soon cut to sixty and, in fact, the number has varied somewhat according to the national financial situation and local circumstances.

One of the great problems was the relationship between the PHLS and hospitals. It seemed a waste of manpower for those laboratories sited in hospitals—and today the vast majority are so sited—not to carry out the bacteriology for the hospital as well as public health work. In addition, there is little incentive for a bacteriologist to work without seeing patients and treating their infections (the general tendency among laboratory doctors has changed during my career and a hospital haematologist will today expect to see and treat patients with blood diseases, leaving most of the laboratory work to non-medical laboratory staff). Thus a compromise has had to be made and, although still nominally primarily directed towards public health bacteriology, many PHLS bacteriologists find that only about 10 per cent of their work has a bearing on public health and the rest is purely clinical bacteriology.

The laboratory services of the National Health Service, i.e. the hospital laboratories, have never been one integrated service so that reference laboratories are not common; thus the reference facilities of the PHLS are frequently made use of by hospital bacteriologists.

A plethora of epidemiologists

Until 1977 the Department of Health and Social Security (DHSS) employed epidemiologists who could visit areas where epidemics were taking place in the interests of the Department itself. By then the MOH had disappeared, to be replaced by the Community Physician, one of whom, the Medical Officer (Environmental Health) was responsible, among other things, for epidemiology. This meant that too large a number of people might be involved in the investigation of an outbreak; they might include: the Director of the local Public Health Laboratory; the local Medical Officer (Environmental Health); the Environmental Health Officer of the local authority; an epidemiologist from the PHLS headquarters; an epidemiologist from the DHSS; and, in cases involving zoonoses, a local veterinary officer.

This would obviously become a matter of too many people being involved. However, the situation was eased a little in 1977, when it was decided that the PHLS should be responsible for 'national' epidemiology and the Communicable Diseases Surveillance Centre was set up at the PHLS at Colindale. This body is responsible for collating material for the *Summary of Weekly Returns* and also for providing epidemiologists to work on outbreaks in other areas.

Thus, in spite of efforts made to eradicate it, we possess in England and Wales one of the finest services for the control of infection and the envy of many countries. As an example, the number of virus laboratories for the population they deal with is greater in Britain than in any other country. And the service arose more or less by accident!

An example of the efficiency of the system is provided by the botulism outbreak of 1989, described in Chapter 9.

The control of infection by means of vaccination

In Chapter 3 we saw how Edward Jenner introduced an efficient and safe method of preventing smallpox by vaccination and how Louis Pasteur did him the honour of using the term 'vaccination' for his method of protecting people against rabies. Since then vaccination has proved to be the most efficient single method for the prevention of those infectious diseases that are amenable to its use. In fact, when a 'new' disease such as AIDS appears, the first reaction is, 'Can a vaccine against it be produced?'

The end of the nineteenth and the beginning of the twentieth centuries marked the heyday of discovery of bacterial vaccines. Vaccines against cholera, typhoid, plague and other infections were introduced but the battle was not without its casualties. For instance, in Malkawal in India, nineteen persons receiving Haffkine's plague vaccine died of tetanus. This tragedy was later echoed in the Cutter Incident and the Lubeck Disaster, described in Chapters 6 and 8 respectively.

Soon after the First World War Calmette and Guérin succeeded in producing their non-pathogenic tubercle bacillus (BCG) and, after a certain number of trials and investigations, it began to play an important part as a vaccine for the prevention of tuberculosis.

Attempts to control virus diseases by vaccination included the pioneer procedures mentioned above, as well as vaccination against smallpox and rabies. Yellow fever vaccine was produced by growing the virus in chick embryos or mouse brain but other viruses had to wait until tissue culture methods had been introduced in the late 1940s. This technique rapidly produced a harvest of vaccines, including those against poliomyelitis, measles, mumps, rubella and influenza. A vaccine against whooping cough was introduced in the mid 1950s and one against hepatitis B a few years after the discovery of the virus. Attempts to produce vaccines against all types of meningococci are still in progress.

Vaccines have changed the face of infectious disease in the West. Smallpox has been eradicated using a vaccine little different from that used by Jenner and Jesty; poliomyelitis has been virtually eradicated, as has been diphtheria, although the latter was allowed to flourish much longer than it should have done in Britain. In the USA measles and rubella have been brought under control; but a different approach to rubella vaccination and poor uptake of measles vaccination have meant that Britain has not been as successful in eradicating these diseases.

Disadvantages of vaccines

All vaccines carry some risk so that one should think twice before undergoing one that is not really necessary. I have seen two deaths in patients undergoing totally unnecessary typhoid vaccination and recently heard of a death following a cholera vaccination in an allergic patient. However, it is more often wise to undergo than not to undergo vaccination.

The possibility of live polio vaccine reverting to type has already been mentioned, with the suggestion that unvaccinated parents should be vaccinated at the same time as the child. Smallpox vaccination was always fairly unpleasant and carried about a one in 100,000 risk of causing encephalitis. For this reason it was preferable to 'ring vaccinate'—that is, vaccinate only contacts of a smallpox patient—rather than to undertake mass vaccination of the whole population. Whooping cough vaccine obtained for itself a bad name some years ago as a cause of brain damage. Recent large surveys have failed to produce any dramatic evidence on the subject but, a bad name having been attached to the procedure, both parents and medical staff still approach the procedure with unfounded suspicion.

The efficiency of vaccines

Efficiency varies. Vaccination against measles, poliomyelitis, yellow fever and diphtheria are very protective and can be up to 100 per cent effective. Typhoid vaccines vary in the degree of protection, which depends also on the size of the dose received (that is, the number of typhoid bacteria swallowed). The efficiency of influenza vaccine is said to vary from nil to 90 per cent and obviously depends on closeness of antigenic resemblance between the influenza A strain in the vaccine and that causing the epidemic. Even with a vaccine of only moderate protective value, vaccination is worthwhile because of the large numbers of people involved.

Diseases in which the offending organisms do not enter the body proper, but remain in the intestinal canal, such as dysentery, salmonella (other than typhoid or paratyphoid) and cholera, are difficult to protect against by vaccination as only small amounts of antibody find their way into the gut. Thus, the cholera vaccine is probably the least useful we have.

Vaccine therapy

For about the first half of this century it was often the practice to use vaccination, not only for the prevention of epidemic diseases but also for the *treatment* of boils, sinusitis and a large number of nonspecific conditions, not all of which might be infectious in nature. A swab was taken from the affected site (or, often, from the nose or throat); any organisms grown would be purified, grown in bulk and killed by heat. Suspensions of these organisms were then injected into the patients, some of whom recovered from their original condition. As a student and young doctor, I well remember the advertising on tube trains of a proprietary 'vaccine' to be taken by mouth; the fact that the stomach acid would destroy the organisms in the 'vaccine' seemed beside the point.

Reasons for poor uptake of vaccination in Britain

Britain lags behind other countries of Europe and behind the USA in the percentage of children vaccinated with the basic vaccines (measles, polio, rubella, diphtheria, tetanus and whooping cough), although targets of 90 per cent uptake in primary immunization rates were set for Europe by 1990.

In December 1988, a man in his sixties and with no history of poliomyelitis vaccination developed the infection while on holiday in Tunisia. He became paralysed in all limbs and needed mechanical ventilation. This illustrates the need for vaccination before travelling to areas where infectious diseases are more common than in Britain. It also illustrates the need to maintain a high proportion of immune people in the population. We have seen that many people can become infected with the poliovirus without illness; the fact that a holidaymaker contracted the infection with symptoms suggests that some at least must have contracted the disease without symptoms and imported the virus duty-free; a low proportion of vaccinated people in the 'home' population would render it likely that such imported infections might well be transmitted to susceptibles after the patient's return home.

Here are some of the reasons for failure to vaccinate in Britain:

1. *Public perception*. Vaccination saves more lives than, say, heart surgery; but the latter is far more glamorous both for the surgeon and the hospital or health district. There is little publicity for a 90 per cent vaccine uptake but a detached finger sewn back in place gets nationwide coverage.
2. *Complacency*. The absence of cases of poliomyelitis or diphtheria pushes out of the mind the efforts needed to eradicate and keep eradicated these diseases.
3. *Abnormal views of normality*. Many parents regard measles (and to a lesser extent, whooping cough) inevitable and 'natural' diseases of childhood. Only parents of the small number of children killed or handicapped by these diseases remain impressed by their importance.
4. *Cowardice*. When parents fear complications from vaccinations, especially those for whooping cough, medical and nursing staff rarely have the courage to attempt to persuade them, knowing full well that

should anything go wrong they would be blamed; an old book of mine on cardiology lays down the precept that no physician should make decisions founded only on his own selfish interests.

There is a great need for much better education of both the public and medical and nursing staff on the importance of vaccination in a modern commercial and industrial nation.

Vaccination in the Third World

If vaccination is important in a modern commercial and industrial country, it is a thousandfold more so in the Third World. I have indicated elsewhere this need but would emphasize it by repeating some figures: there are nearly 3,000,000 children who die, 200,000 who are paralysed and 150,000 who are blinded by diseases that can be prevented by vaccination.

Individual lifestyle and the control of infection

At the end of his excellent book, *Man, Microbe and Malady*, published in 1940, Dr John Drew writes:

> Our duty as individuals is to conserve our bodily and mental resistance by good living and clean thinking, to protect our children by careful upbringing and the intelligent use of the preventive measures that medical science provides and to take care that we do not spread any infection that we may have contracted among our fellow-countrymen.

If this had not been published in wartime, the last word might have been 'fellow human beings'. However, there is little to add to that exhortation and what follows is merely an updating.

Infection and drugs of addiction

I have perhaps been over fanciful in my choice of these drugs; many would disagree about a couple. However, overindulgence in any of them will lower a person's resistance to infections of various kinds.

Tobacco. Although cancer of the lung is the most dramatic of the wages of tobacco smoking, a commoner one is the chronic smoker's cough (a performance beautifully executed by Polly, our parrot—see Chapter 8). This is caused by irritation of the mucous membrane together with an over-secretion of mucus. This has to be coughed up, leading to damage of the linings of the air passages. This weakened state of the respiratory tract allows infection by organisms not normally sufficiently dangerous to cause infection. A smoker's cough can also mask chronic tuberculous infection.

Alcohol. Over use of alcohol lets in infection in a variety of ways. Damage to the liver reduces the production of antibody and other factors necessary to immunity. There is also the possibility of inhaling vomit during a drunken stupor; this can cause severe pneumonia at best and rapid death from asphyxia at worst. People unconscious as a result of alcohol excesses are also liable to suffer from exposure, following which infection, especially respiratory, is likely to occur.

Food. This is a drug of addiction to some. Being overweight renders one susceptible to infection, especially respiratory infection. Studies among populations on the edge of starvation and in animals suggest that infection is best resisted by those whose diet is slightly below what is considered the optimum. On the other hand, starvation of course frequently ends in death from infection, as we have seen in recent terrible famines.

Recognized drugs of addiction. Drugs such as cocaine and morphia soon reduce the body's resistance and infection follows. This may be a local infection, caused by dirty needles, or a generalized infection, such as septicaemia. Subjects dying from drug addiction usually actually die from associated infection. In addition to these general infections, two fairly recently-emerged infections are particularly liable to occur in intravenous drug addicts. Hepatitis B, discovered in 1968, was found to have caused many cases of jaundice following blood transfusion. This is no longer the case, as all samples of blood are tested for antibody to the virus before issuing. However, it can easily be spread from subject to subject when syringes and needles are shared for the purpose of injecting drugs. A very similar approach is taken by another recently discovered virus—the Human Immunodeficiency Virus (HIV) that causes AIDS. Although HIV infection is chiefly through male homosexual activity, most women suffering from the infection, in Britain at least, are those who have contracted it from others by shared syringes in the context of drug addiction.

Sex. This, like food, is generally looked upon as a necessity of life but, for some, it can become addictive. The divinity in charge of human enjoyment seems to have been engaged for a long time in a programme aimed at spoiling the enjoyment of sex. Years ago the wages of promiscuity were the 'old-fashioned' sexually transmitted diseases of syphilis and gonorrhoea. When antibiotics emerged it appeared that both of these diseases could be treated successfully at last, so that the only hazard to sex, illicit or otherwise, was unwanted pregnancy. Then the contraceptive pill came along and the outlook seemed fine. Then, in quick succession, appeared two serious infections spread by sex: hepatitis B and HIV infection (leading to AIDS).

A worker already quoted has suggested that HIV infection follows abnormal sex—either too much (as in prostitutes) or the wrong type (as in homosexuals). Control of these diseases necessitates a change of lifestyle in the person at risk—the use of condoms, monogamy or the abandonment of penetrative sex completely (See Chapter 7).

I do not intend to reiterate the many recommendations on infection control made over the years, including such matters as personal hygiene, food hygiene, good hospital practice, efficient sewage disposal and the availability of a supply of pure drinking water, as most have been dealt with earlier; but they *are* most important factors, together with those just mentioned, in enabling everybody to play his part in the control of infection. The words of Dr Drew quoted earlier should be remembered.

FIFTEEN

Infection in the Future

Prediction is not difficult providing one sticks to the two limits of the future: tomorrow, for instance, will be very like today but, in order to court popularity, it may be painted a little more rosy; and when the universe finally drags to an end (and entropy rules OK) there is no longer any comment worth making. As far as the rest of the future is concerned the only true prediction to be made is that the majority of predictions will prove inaccurate.

False and true predictions

If an intelligent being living three thousand million years ago was told that in the oceans of the planet Earth four or so small molecules had got together to form a larger one capable of limited self-replication, he would probably react with mild interest; what he would have called life needed much more vigour, and a source of energy, such as radioactivity, would be needed in order to give rise to what he would think of as living beings.

If, many millions of years later, he or his descendants were to hear that some of these lowly Earth molecules had managed to manufacture a green pigment that unlocked the energy of the sun for them, he would have been very interested and most likely predicted the eventual appearance of large motile, airbreathing green creatures; he would probably not have taken into account the phenomenon of predation.

During the courses of the ancient civilizations, the manipulation of infection was left in the hands of the deities, who used it chiefly as a weapon of punishment. The human prophets confined themselves mainly to political and historical matters and, because such early works on these subjects were usually written retrospectively, they were usually correct.

In the Middle Ages, we have to look to astrologers for forecasts of the future. While Martin Luther shared the opinion that all pestilences were brought on the people by evil spirits, an astrologer, at the ripe old age of 108, forecast that, when Saturn and Jupiter were in conjunction (and with other portents), plague would appear within two years; the plague would be so severe that it would even carry off cats and dogs (plague was such a common visitor at this time that prophesying it was rather like forecasting an earth tremor in San Francisco).

If, by 'prediction', we also mean explaining the cause of a disease before scientific proof of the theory has been obtained, then we can include such well-known theories as the origin of malaria from 'bad air' and the effects of the influences of the planets in causing influenza.

Among so many predictions, some had to be right. In 1719, for instance, Benjamin Marten believed that tuberculosis was contagious and suggested that the disease was due to 'some certain species of small Animalcules or wonderfully minute living Creatures that, by their peculiar Shape or Disagreeable Parts, are inimical to our natures'.

Some personal views of the future

This chapter, happily one of the shortest, represents some of my personal views of the future. As I am neither a politician nor a philosopher (except in the very common sense), many will find some of them naive.

Perhaps the best way to play the Old Moore is to consider first some of the infections mentioned in the Introduction as being topical at present, then deal with other problems of the West and suggest an approach to their solution. After that, the greater problems of the Third World will be considered, a situation where imagination is needed to conceive a solution.

Some topical infections

The formation of the welfare state has caused every citizen to expect, if not to receive, complete immunity from infectious diseases and the State is regarded as the paid agent of the people in ensuring for them this immunity.

We have already seen that it was earlier thought that the two main weapons to be used against infection were antibiotics and vaccination. If antibiotics have been found to be a promise half fulfilled, then vaccination must be a gift only half accepted. It is available to all; yet, with the exceptions of diphtheria and poliomyelitis, vaccination rates in the population are still not sufficiently high enough to eradicate the disease which vaccination is designed to protect against.

AIDS. Widespread advice on this subject already seems to be reaping some reward. Although some of the people to whom propaganda has been directed seem not to absorb it, a marked alteration of the sexual habits of many, both heterosexual and homosexual but more particularly among homosexuals, has taken place over the last few years, with a reduction of promiscuity and greater use of condoms. I believe that this change in habits will reduce the growth of AIDS over the next few years. Search for a vaccine or a curative therapeutic substance will be carried on, on both financial and humanitarian grounds; I rather fancy that the search for antiviral drugs will lead to the discovery of one suitable for treating HIV infection before a suitable vaccine has been elaborated.

Hepatitis B. This infection has been overshadowed by HIV infection, which it superficially resembles, but it is still an important cause of illness. In this case an excellent vaccine exists but, because of the complexity of its manufacture, it is very expensive. This vaccine is obtained from the blood of heavy carriers of the hepatitis B virus; hence, expensive precautions against the infection of the manufacturing staff and against the risk of producing a batch containing live virus render the price of the finished product almost prohibitive. New and cheaper ways of producing a vaccine will be used successfully; these may include the synthesizing of some of the peptides (strings of amino acids) that occur naturally on the surface of the virus or inserting part or all of one of the genes of the virus into a chromosome of a bacterium or yeast; as the organism grows it produces hepatitis B antigen in large amounts and very cheaply; these two methods, once set up, do not involve any infectious material. In Africa the production of a cheap hepatitis B vaccine would be a godsend.

Influenza. There has been no major change in the genetic make-up of the influenza A virus for many years and it may be that such a change will not occur. The world's influenza surveillance system is very efficient and, if a major variant *should* arise, it is likely that the new strain will be introduced into an up-to-date vaccine quickly enough to protect most populations at risk. It is most unlikely that outbreaks on the scale of that of 1918 will ever occur again.

Legionnaire's disease. This is an example of an infection caused by an organism that can exist in the environment without needing a human or animal host, an attribute it shares with the organisms causing botulism, gas gangrene and tetanus. Thus, it would seem difficult to eradicate it by vaccination as in the cases of smallpox and poliomyelitis. We have to depend upon correct maintenance of the environment to remain free from this infection and legislation in this direction will be more valuable than most. It is essential to have good design and regular cleaning in all situations where water that has been static for a while is sprayed into the environment; cooling towers, air conditioning plant and shower heads must be the subject of constant scrutiny. We must always be on the outlook for other 'spraying' mechanisms that might induce further outbreaks.

Listeria infections. The organism that causes this infection is also free living, being found in fields, mouldy fodder, birds and the stools of animals and humans. It is an organism of very low pathogenicity and appears to attack only those with reduced immunity and pregnant women. It is found in various foods but its presence in the environment is probably of more importance than its detection in foodstuffs. However, it can cause death, especially of unborn children, and infections due to this organism seem to be increasing. The only advice that can be given is for expectant mothers to stick to home cooking and to wash their own salads; the presence of the organism in the environment will probably render this advice of little value.

Rubella. As a result of the use of the new measles, mumps and rubella vaccine, congenital rubella infection will be expected eventually to disappear; but it will not be before many years that the full impact of the new vaccination programme will be felt. In the meantime, because both boys and girls are to be vaccinated, the number of infections in children will fall; the number of contacts available to pregnant women will then be reduced and the incidence of congenital rubella will fall gradually, after about five or six years, with the full effect in up to thirty years.

Salmonella infections. Although these were with us before the Second World War, it is only since then that we have enjoyed the presence of a vast variety of different strains and that we allowed these organisms to get into our livestock through contaminated feeding stuffs. We knew that ducks harboured these organisms in their ovaries and produced eggs that were encapsulated agents of infection. This has now happened to some flocks (batteries?) of hens. It is essential that we return to clean livestock. In the case of hens it is feasible to get rid of those with ovarian infection with compensation but, with larger animals, it is a different matter. It is to be hoped that the Department of Agriculture will encourage breeders of livestock to rear salmonella-free animals in the way that tuberculosis-free herds are maintained, keeping them apart from other herds and subjecting them to regular veterinary inspection and using only monitored feed; more direct methods of marketing should be adopted so that uninfected animals are not herded with infected ones in vans and pens. In this way I believe that, in time, the root source of salmonella infection will be eradicated and the many hygenic practices advocated for food preparation will not carry such a great responsibility for the avoidance of infection as they do today.

Other infections in the West

The impossibility of the task of predicting the future of infection can be deduced from the events of the last twenty-five years. We have seen a constant upsurge of 'new' infections, which range between the exotic (Marburg fever, Ebola fever, Lassa fever) and the serious (hepatitis B, AIDS, Legionnaire's disease). In exchange, we have lost smallpox completely and practically lost poliomyelitis and diphtheria. Meningitis appears to have increased in incidence but, as soon as the cost and effort seem worthwhile, a vaccine against the commonest type will be available. A recent newspaper article suggested that a cure for the common cold is on the way, but this has been promised many times before.

A new and more efficient vaccine for whooping cough will be devised and the question of the role of this vaccine in the cause of brain damage will be elucidated. (When using a substance that will be administered to perhaps millions of subjects, it is only by giving it to large numbers that rare instances causing damage can be quantified. For instance, it has been estimated that one in 100,000 people vaccinated against smallpox developed serious illness; it was necessary to vaccinate well over 100,000 to discover this. Thus, in 1961–2 there were twenty-six deaths from smallpox in Britain with twelve deaths caused by vaccination; this led to the abandonment in 1971 of vaccination soon after birth.)

Hospital infections are likely to continue in the near future; an end to the present understaffing of hospitals would allow a greater interest in methods of combating this form of infection.

The emergence of new organisms

Some of the 'new' infectious diseases have been caused by 'old' organisms 'coming out of retirement'; organisms of the legionnella group were isolated from an infection as long ago as 1947. In other cases, what were suspected to be diseases in their own right have been separated from those causing similar infections by new laboratory techniques; thus, long before the Second World War it was believed that there was more than one organism capable of causing jaundice, but this was not confirmed until the work of Blumberg and the full description of the hepatitis B virus.

New variations of 'old' viruses appear from time to time and it has been suggested that new serotypes of influenza A viruses may occur through the crossing of a human strain (to which most of the population had become immune) with an animal strain; the contribution of the animal strain was a new coat, unrecognizable by the immune systems of those immune to the human strain, while the human strain contributed the ability to take over the metabolism of the cell that had been invaded and to cause it to produce more virus. This process of 'crossing' of different strains of a virus is easily carried out in the laboratory by infecting tissue culture with two closely related strains of the same virus.

The emergence of really new viruses is always a matter of speculation and, in considering the future, we have to consider how viruses new to ourselves have emerged. In Chapter 11, I suggested that the Third World constituted a vast laboratory where the viruses, at present infecting animals, tried their hand at infecting humans, often with signal success. The origin of HIV is shrouded in mystery, if only because indications are that it was about long before the original cases of 1981. The presence of related viruses – HIV-2 affecting humans and SIV infecting monkeys as well as strains infecting other animals – suggests that it has been evolving for many years. A number of ancestor viruses have been suggested for HIV, including that causing African horse disease, but there is little evidence to link any of these to it.

It seems only too certain that similar viruses, with their substrains, will emerge regularly in the future, but it is doubtful if any will pose such problems as the virus causing AIDS. Some years ago it was said that the deepfreezers of most virus laboratories were bursting with specimens of new viruses waiting to be identified. These are probably not important; it is the serious disease whose cause must be sought that is important, not the new virus waiting to have a disease attached to it.

Infection and cancer

Accessory genetic material in the cell

It has long been known that certain viruses are able to cause cancer in animals and some also in humans. The way in which they do this is complex and not fully understood and involves some consideration of molecular biology.

When I discussed the way bacteria became resistant to antibiotics as a result of a change in the nature of the genetic material in the nucleus, it was obvious that the one organism that had undergone this change would need to multiply for many generations before the culture was predominantly antibiotic resistant. There are other methods whereby organisms become resistant.

As well as the nucleus, many bacterial cells carry little collections of genetic material in the cytoplasm, known as plasmids. (See Figure 15.1.) Plasmids are not necessary for the cell's multiplication but they do give it certain new abilities. One of the first discovered is known as F and bacteria possessing this plasmid are able to conjugate, i.e. two come together and mix their genetic material; this is a primitive form of sex. Other plasmids, known as R factors are able to show the bacterium how to make enzymes to inactivate antibiotics. These factors are *infectious*, i.e. they can be released into the culture medium where they can infect bacteria previously without them. This is a matter of practical importance, because a patient may be infected by a strain of *Salm. typhi* sensitive to, say, chloramphenicol. Within the bowel of that patient may

Figure 15.1 A plasmid within a cell

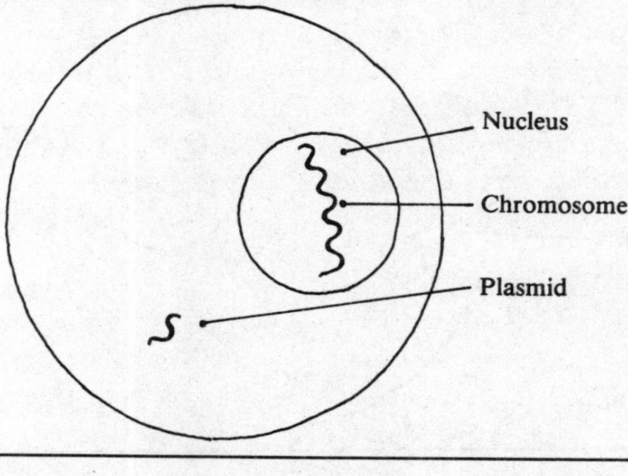

be coliform organisms containing plasmids of the R variety making those organisms resistant to chloromphenicol. Also within the bowel these plasmids can be released and passed to the typhoid bacilli; thus, the patient's stools will contain typhoid bacilli resistant to chloramphenicol and further infections with this strain of typhoid bacillus will be difficult to treat.

As well as plasmids, bacteria may be invaded by bacteriophages. (See Figure 15.2.) These small viruses attach themselves to the bacterial wall and inject their genetic material into the cell. Within the cell this material may do several things; it may multiply and eventually kill the bacterium; it may remain in the cytoplasm doing nothing or it may become inserted into the strand of genetic material constituting the bacterium's nucleus. (See Figure 15.3.) Genetic material conveys information and the new material present in the nucleus may give the bacterium more abilities. An example of this is in the case of the diphtheria bacillus. As we have seen, this organism multiplies in the patient's throat and produces a toxin that can prove fatal. Now the only diphtheria bacilli that produce toxin are those that have been infected by a certain bacteriophage which has become integrated into its nucleus. (See Figure 15.4.) If the bacteriophage is got rid of, the diphtheria no longer produces toxin and is quite harmless to man.

It is difficult to trace the evolution and relationship between plasmids and bacteriophages. Are they more or less the same entity? Did they evolve from detached bits of genetic material from cells? To what extent are the genetic contents of our cells derived from plasmids or bacterio-

Figure 15.2 Bacterium and bacteriophage

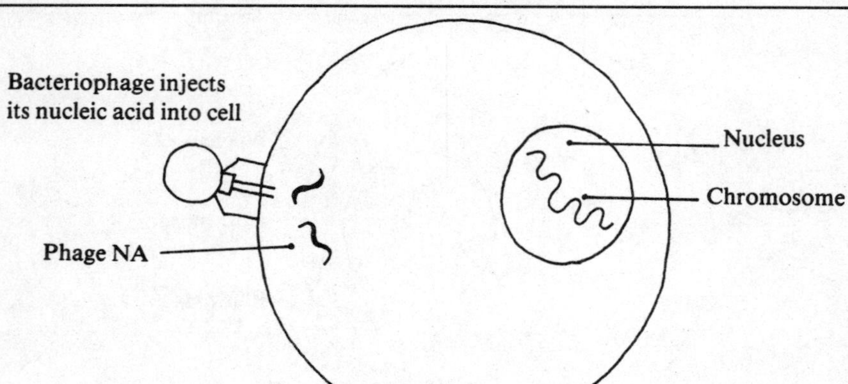

Figure 15.3 Phage nucleic acid is integrated into cell's chromosome

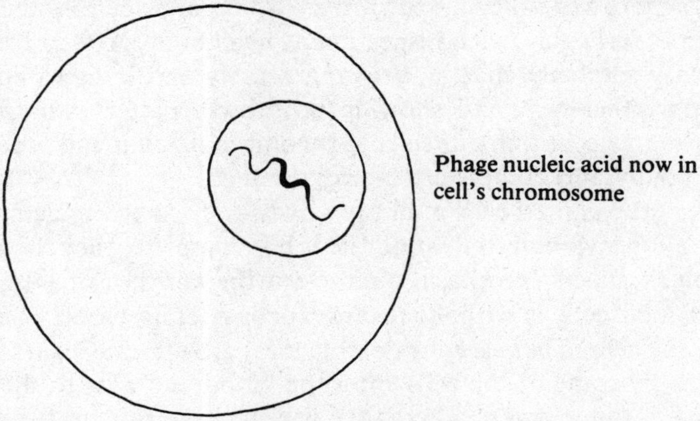

phages? Can these small structures 'carry' genetic material from one species of cell to another, to be permanently included in the nucleus? These considerations show how complex must be the origin of our genetic material, perhaps containing much genetic debris that has drifted in from outside sources, some playing no part, some useful and some positively dangerous.

Figure 15.4 Diphtheria toxin production

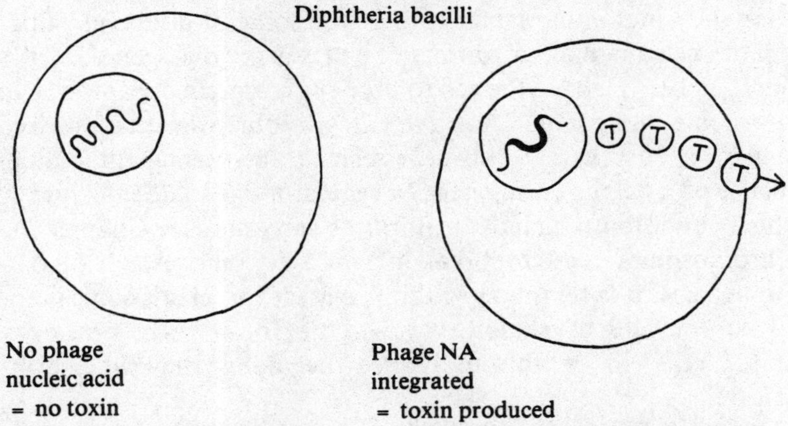

What is cancer?

When cells from a monkey kidney are grown in tissue culture they first grow in an orderly way, each respecting its neighbour. After a few sub-cultures they suddenly change, growing rapidly and indiscriminately, lying across other cells and showing no growth pattern whatsoever. What has happened is that one cell has become malignant and proceeded to grow rapidly and completely unprogrammed.

In the healthy animal cells multiply slowly and, when replacing dead cells or healing a wound, only until the job is complete; they then cease to multiply. Cancers (neoplasms) represent the antithesis to this. The growth of their cells is without regard to considerations of space and neighbouring cells. There is considerable local growth causing a tumour and frequently some of the cells enter the blood and pass to the liver, brain, lung or other organ, where they continue to grow, as if released from their social obligations by some Sorcerer's Apprentice. They block blood vessels, press out by sheer weight the vital cells in the organs affected and eventually kill the patient.

Figure 15.5 Genes on human chromosome

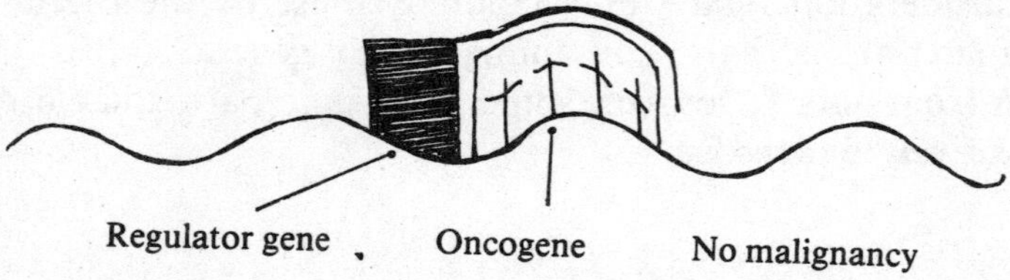

Oncogenes

Among the genes in human cells there are some of doubtful value; one group of such a malignant variety of genes is the oncogenes. If allowed to function they instruct the cell to produce a protein capable of causing it to become malignant. Thus, we carry in our own cells the seeds of malignancy. Fortunately, this gene seems to be permanently under the influence of a neighbouring gene, a regulatory gene. (See Figure 15.5.) In some conditions, such as in Burkitt's sarcoma (see Chapter 5), bits of chromosomes tend to break off and become attached to other chromosomes; it is tempting to think that, if the break comes between an oncogene and a regulatory gene, the former will be no longer inhibited but will be able to induce the malignancy we see in this condition.

This rather long preamble leads to a consideration of how viruses cause malignancy. Many of the viruses implicated in the generation of cancer are the retroviruses which contain RNA in their chromosomes (HIV is a retrovirus but is not carcenogenic). These retroviruses contain oncogenes similar to those in animal cell nuclei; this indicates that these viruses have, in the remote past, 'hijacked' that portion of the cell's genetic material containing the oncogene, leaving behind the bit containing the regulator. Thus, entry into a suitable cell might lead to it mediating the carcinogenic protein. (See Figure 15.6.)

I have gone into the question of viruses causing malignancy because I feel that work on this subject will, in the not-too-distant future, clarify our minds on the subject of the causation of cancer and, it is hoped, lead to prevention of at least some forms.

The future of Third World infection

I have already tried to convey the enormous importance of infection in the Third World and to suggest that the great differences between the Third World and the West are almost entirely due to poverty. Many improvements in the situation could be made by the injection of sufficient money, although this is not the ultimate solution.

Malaria. This could be much reduced in incidence. Although some degree of immunity develops in people constantly exposed to infection, it is often at the expense of previous chronic infection; immigrants from malarial areas to the West must remember that this immunity tends to wane after a year or so if they are considering revisiting their home country. The chances of producing a vaccine are, at present, not too hopeful and, in any case, it would be preferable to go to the source of the problem and eradicate the mosquito responsible. Attempts should

Figure 15.6 Genes on a retrovirus

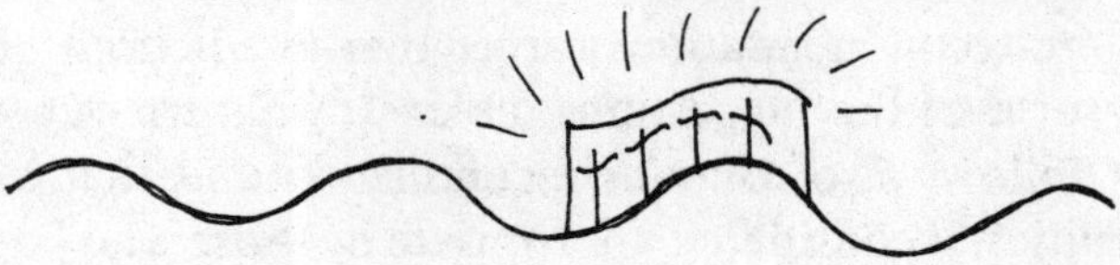

No regulator gene Oncogene fully active Malignancy

If there is no regulator gene to repress the oncogene, the cell is likely to become malignant.

be made to drain swamps and treat with larvicides any stagnant water remaining.

Trypanosomiasis—African. Drugs may be used for prophylaxis but more drastic methods are needed for near eradication. In the case of the Gambian variety, where man is the chief reservoir, the seeking out and treating of human cases is important. Reduction of wild game might reduce the incidence of the Rhodesian type but, both because of conservational interests and the fact that the parasite would probably move over to infect domestic animals, this action is, perhaps, not recommended. More important is the clearing of bush or forest beside streams.

Trypanosomiasis—South American. The provision of dwellings with smooth-plastered walls is practically all that is needed to remove the reduviid bug and, with it, the majority of South American trypanosomiasis. Perhaps the countries of South America will be relieved of their debts and spend their money, perhaps earned through their own delayed industrial revolution, in the rehousing of their people.

Liver carcinoma. In many parts of Africa, where the incidence of carriers of the hepatitis B virus is 25 per cent or more, the incidence of liver cancer is huge compared with that in the rest of the world; there seems little doubt that the virus causes the cancer and it seems desirable that a cheap hepatitis B vaccine should be developed and used to vaccinate newborn babies or children who are not carriers in that part of the world. Although the results would not be felt for thirty years or so, there is little doubt that the situation would be eventually greatly improved.

The problem of the Third World

All the above are recommendations rather than predictions but it is to be hoped that some of the suggestions, at least, will turn out to be prophesies. What follows also contains recommendations that it is hoped will come to fruition if considered appropriate by those who know better than I do.

The actions recommended above all involve the spending of vast amounts of money and the sources of such money have to be considered. In Britain, whenever a famine or similar disaster in the Third World is reported on television news programmes (radio had and has much less impact), it is the signal for prominent people to organize events designed to provide large amounts of money; food and other essentials are sent with as little delay to the affected area so that fewer die than might have done. The nation enjoys a comfortable feeling of self-esteem and then turns back to its more usual activities until a further famine is reported. This intermittent action is, of course, better than none at all, but not as useful as a constant supply of money to be used with common sense and joined with other ideas.

It seems essential that an international body be set up to look into the question of making conditions in the Third World more comparable with those existing in the West; this could be linked to the United Nations Organization, its medical activities worked out through the World Health Organization. It could be financed through contributions from western nations, perhaps, in the future, from what is saved from their military budgets following the recent outbreak of goodwill between the superpowers.

Money is not enough

It is already being recognized that a supply of food and shelter during a period of famine or drought is only a holding operation. Next year or the year after the situation will recur. Attempts are being made by relief organizations to make the local people more self-sufficient, to provide sources of water unaffected by drought and to arm them with more efficient tools and more suitable crop plants.

This, in itself, is a move in the right direction but little permanent can be done until the Third World enjoys its own Industrial Revolution. Before this can be done two other goals must be reached. The first is a limitation of population; contraception of one sort or another must be made popular in the Third World so that a man no longer hangs on to the philosophy that, the more children he has, the better he will be looked after in his old age (however, it must be said that many experts believe that a stable economy will, itself, alter this philosophy without the need for outside pressure in the matter). The second goal is the bringing of some kind of organization to the Third World. This is a complex matter; it involves both physical matters (such as road building so that all inhabitants are able to reach centres of civilization quickly) and also more tenuous matters (such as the instillation of a sort of civic responsibility in all, especially the relatively powerful, and the elimination of tribalism and other causes of conflict). An end to apartheid is implicit in these proposals.

Once the correct scenario has been reached, it will be necessary to introduce suitable industries to boost the wealth of the nation. This is a difficult matter because the setting up of such industries will not be to the West's advantage, as we have seen when former Third World nations (or at least Second World nations) such as Japan, Korea, Taiwan and Singapore have set up their own manufacturing industries. The setting up of even more industries in even more countries will tend to even out gross national incomes so that the West will lose out to the advantage of the Third World.

These arguments may seem a little naive to the experts, but must provide a skeleton of any successful scheme to bring infection in the Third World down to what we would consider a reasonable level.

Let us hope that some, at least, of these suggestions become predictions.

Will infection ever be eradicated?

The answer is a definite 'No'. While there is any degree of variety of life on Earth there will be organisms to make use of most of it. Predation is one of the ways evolution works and life is a very plastic material. If all the food poisoning and dysentery bacteria were suddenly magically killed, I am sure that one of the more entrepreneurial of the 'good' organisms in the bowel would alter its lifestyle to replace them. Bacteria can live in many sorts of environments and will fill any niche in which they can possibly grow by adapting themselves to the conditions there.

In addition, completely to eradicate bacteria would be hard on the ruminants who depend upon them to derive energy from the grass of the field; gut bacteria in other animals probably produce small amounts of vitamin-like substances that are needed for the well being of those animals, so that bacteria play a positive and helpful role in many circumstances.

Thus we cannot afford to eradicate all bacteria even if it were possible and, if we could eradicate only the pathogens, certain of the non-pathogens would evolve to become pathogenic. The best we can hope for is to control the causes of the most serious infectious diseases and hope that the remainder will remain interesting but relatively harmless.

Index

The Smallest Enemy

Typography by Little Red Cloud
Cover design by Frances Ross
Figures and illustrations by Harriet Duncan
based on the author's drawings
Composed by Colset Private Limited of Singapore
in Compugraphic 11/13 point English Times
Printed and bound by
Billing & Sons of Worcester, England
on Publisher's Antique Wove paper
Production supervised by Grant Shipcott